you are what you eat

you are what you eat

80 simple, healthy family recipes

Foreword by
Dr Amir Khan & Trisha Goddard

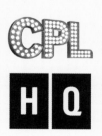

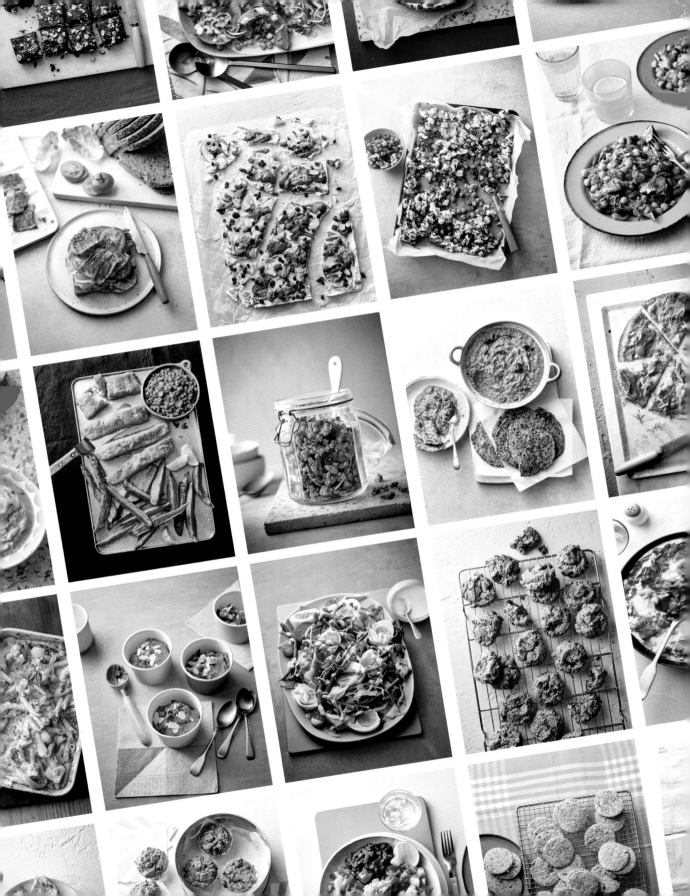

Contents

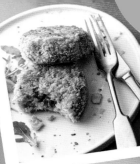
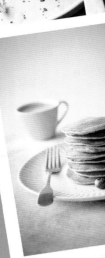
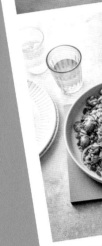
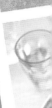
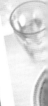

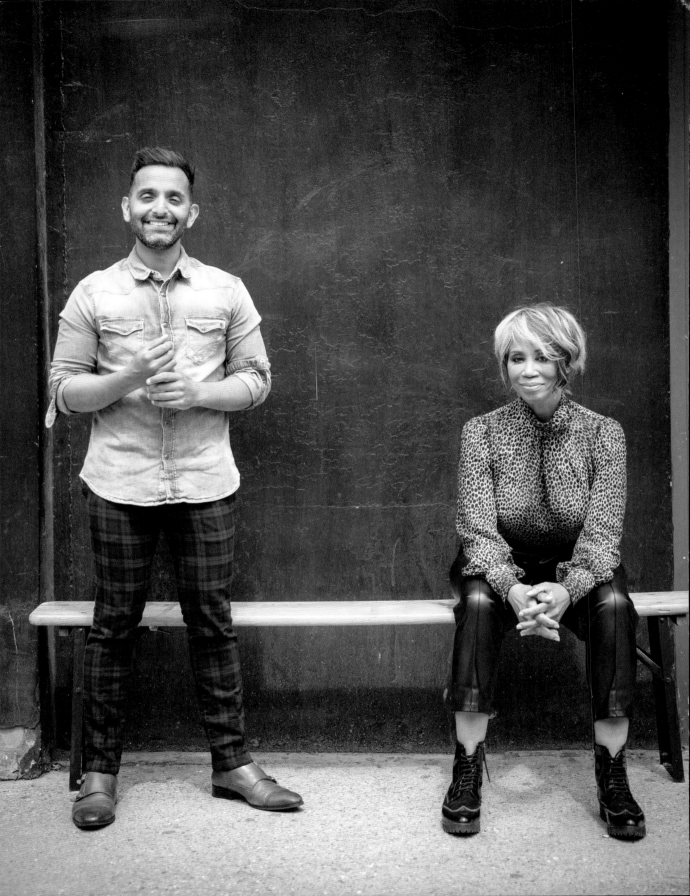

FOREWORD

Dr Amir Khan & Trisha Goddard

Having good health is central to our happiness as human beings.

Being healthy means different things to different people, but most agree that it should include having optimum physical, mental and social wellbeing – not just the absence of illness.

Our bodies are wonderful, unique things that perform little miracles each day – most of which we are not even aware of! Our body's job is not only to keep us in the best condition it can be so that we can perform our daily tasks at an optimum level, but also to provide the mental stability that is needed to take on day-to-day challenges.

For too long, physical and mental health have been thought of as two very separate entities, but it is impossible to have good health without both body and mind functioning well, and increasingly research is showing us just how intimately the two are linked. Although it can feel like a daunting task, looking after both your physical and mental health every single day is what will keep you happier in the long run.

Think of your body and mind as a machine – they both need fuel to function. Your mind requires fuel in the form of positive relationships with other people and your own self-esteem, but mental health is also impacted by what we eat. Some foods can be detrimental to our mental health, but certain foods have actually been proven to have beneficial effects on our moods.

Our physical bodies need good food in appropriate amounts. A healthy diet isn't just about counting calories – even if you are overweight – but how much nutritional value those calories have. It might seem obvious, but you can actually eat quite a lot of food that is high in nutritional value and not worry about its calorific value.

What are processed foods, and why should you avoid them?

You might have heard a lot about processed foods. This is food that has undergone a change from its natural state or has been industrially processed before it's packaged and sold. This applies to any food you buy – and includes fresh, healthy foods! Ultra- processed foods are the ones to avoid, as these have been linked to weight gain, heart disease and some cancers. They lack nutrients and fibre, so in the list below, go green as much as possible, amber in moderation and restrict the red!

UNPROCESSED OR MINIMALLY PROCESSED FOODS

These are ingredients that have had intervention to get from field to plate, such as trimming, cleaning, freezing or pasteurising for preservation.

Includes fruit, vegetables, milk, meat, lentils, seeds, grains like rice, and eggs. Some ingredients might have been produced with the use of fertilisers or steroids (in the case of meat and dairy), so to avoid consuming these, opt for organic products.

PROCESSED FOODS

These have been through a bit more processing, either to make them last longer or to taste better, and generally this includes adding some salt, oil or sugar.

Includes cheese, bacon, tinned fruit or veg, smoked fish.

ULTRA-PROCESSED FOODS

These have been through a lot more processing, and you can spot these by the long list of ingredients that are on the packet – many of which might have numbers and letters and other things that you've never heard of. These extra ingredients are unnatural preservatives, sweeteners, flavours and colour.

Includes processed meat such as sausages and hamburgers, breakfast cereals and cereal bars, fizzy drinks, cakes, chocolate, ice cream, ready meals.

Ultra-processed foods

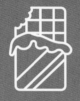

Chocolate

Cake

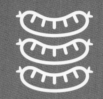

Processed meat

Meal-replacement shakes

Instant soups

Ice cream

Sugary fizzy drinks

Chicken nuggets

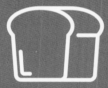

Ice cream

Breakfast cereals or cereal bars

Ready meals, such as pies and pizza

Start as you mean to go on

Once you've completed your food diary, sit down and look at it carefully. Can you identify the 'danger/red foods' and see how much of your diet consists of these? Also look at when you are eating. Is it at regular times of the day? How many times a day? Is most of your food being consumed at mealtimes or as snacks throughout the day and evening? Do you skip meals then make up for these later with a larger meal or more snacks? Eating in an unstructured way can play havoc with your blood-sugar levels, which in turn can affect your energy levels and will have you reaching for sugary foods for a brief and unsustainable boost.

So decide now on a regular eating pattern, because sticking to a routine will also help you to keep you on track with your healthy eating goals. Planning ahead to decide what you will eat and when (see the recipes from page 62 onwards for inspiration) and setting a routine will help you with shopping for your food and keeping to a budget (see the meal planner on page 210), so both your waistline and wallet will benefit.

The important thing to remember when you change your diet is to be positive. Don't see this as banning foods. Instead, think about how you are boosting your intake of delicious, more nutritious food, and how much better you are going to feel by doing this.

The lowdown on snacking

When you're planning your new way of eating, think about how much of your diet is coming from snacks. Snacking in itself is okay, but these little in-between bites need to be small – between 100–150kcals each – and healthy. They should never be a substitute for meals because they are usually too high in calories, fat or sugar and are lower in fibre. Just one evening snack consisting of 80g of popcorn and 1 bag of fruit pastilles adds up to 924kcals and 106g sugar, which is nearly double the recommended daily allowance.

So, swap biscuits, sweets, cakes and muffins for fresh fruit, chopped raw veggies, rice cakes, natural yoghurt with fruit or homemade trail mix. Making your own cookies and cakes also allows you to cut back on the amount of sugar used, or use natural sugar substitutes.

FACT

According to *The Grocer* magazine, 30% of adults in the UK say they skip at least one meal a day in favour of snacking.

Look at the whole picture

It's not just your diet that affects your health and wellbeing; it's important to look at all elements of your current lifestyle that could be impacting your mental and physical health. Here are the key areas that you need to consider:

EXERCISE	Are you getting enough exercise? Keeping active is important for a healthy and strong body and mind and for reducing the risk of health conditions such as heart disease and Type 2 diabetes. If you have a fairly sedentary lifestyle, you need to try to incorporate some form of daily exercise into your routine (see page 52). A healthy diet is also important for exercising because poor nutritional habits will make it harder for your body to reach peak performance – it needs to be supported nutritionally to do what it needs to do.
STRESS	A stressful lifestyle or job could cause you to suffer high blood pressure, poor sleep and anxiety (see page 56). Stress also suppresses the immune system, making you more susceptible to illness. Feeling stressed and under pressure can also lead to emotional eating and overeating, which can lead to obesity.
SLEEP	Lack of sleep or poor-quality sleep can seriously impact your ability to function properly on a daily basis, from feeling a bit slow or fuzzy headed to fighting the urge to reach for unhealthy snacks for an energy boost. Lack of sleep has also been linked to obesity (see page 60).
SMOKING AND ALCOHOL	Are you indulging in these bad habits too often? The impact of smoking on your body is well known; quitting will reduce your risk of heart disease, stroke, cancer and lung disease. Alcohol is linked to numerous serious health conditions, including heart and liver disease, Type 2 diabetes, certain cancers and obesity; drinking alcohol should be kept to a minimum. The recommended limit for men and women is 14 units per week, which equates to 6 pints of average-strength beer or 10 small glasses of wine.

We will explore all these factors in more detail, but for now, consider how your daily life is being impacted in these areas and the way that you are feeling right now. Write down which of these issues feature in your life, and what you'd like to change.

Ditch the junk

You've made the decision to revamp your lifestyle, and the best way to get started is to remove temptation. So, it's time to ditch the junk. If it's not in the kitchen you won't be tempted to eat it, and as you set up new habits, you won't miss it either.

Go through the fridge, freezer and your cupboards and take out everything that doesn't fit with your new, healthier way of eating – that means all processed foods that are full of sugar, salt, fats and additives. If in doubt, check the labels to see if they are green for go (see the table on page 12).

If you hate waste, you could give away some of your foods to neighbours or friends, or even give long-life, unopened packages to food banks, if they are happy to take them. Do not decide to eat them before you get started on your new way of eating; you are just delaying the moment.

Ditch the takeaway menus and dust off your saucepans, or go and buy some shiny new ones. Part of eating healthily is preparing food from scratch, then you'll know exactly what is in everything you eat and you can tailor every meal to your own tastes and nutritional needs (see opposite). Whether you're a novice in the kitchen or a confident chef, there are recipes in this book that are so easy to do, you'll wonder why you didn't start before!

Your new lifestyle starts now. Let's get started!

HEALTHY EATING

So, let's begin with the basics. What should you be eating, and what foods should you be avoiding?

The key to a nutritionally balanced diet is diversity; one that includes all the food groups needed for optimal growth and development and to help reduce the risk of major illnesses like heart disease, diabetes, hypertension, stroke and cancer. Every day you should be aiming to eat from these groups:

1. **Fruit and veg:** This should make up one-third of your daily diet. You might have heard the government advice of eating 5 a day, but general consensus by nutritionists is this isn't enough and we should be looking to have half a plate of veg and salad with each meal, and eat fruit at meals and as snacks.

2. **Starchy foods:** Another third of your diet each day. This includes potatoes, bread, rice, pasta or other starchy carbohydrates.

3. **Dairy or dairy alternatives:** These are important sources of protein, vitamins and minerals such as calcium.

4. **Beans, pulses, fish, eggs and meat:** All are good sources of protein, vitamins and minerals.

In simple terms, we should be looking to increase the amount of nutritious foods we eat and reduce our consumption of those that contain excessive amounts of sugar, 'unhealthy' fats and salt. You can get a headstart on this by simply ditching the junk food and processed food, such as takeaways and ready meals (see page 12), and getting into the kitchen to cook from scratch using fresh ingredients. But while healthy eating means avoiding processed foods, it doesn't apply to all foods that come in a packet – tinned fruit and veg, breads, etc are all good. The big supermarkets and food manufacturers have to display the

Fruit

Fruits are high in nutrients and fibre and relatively low in calories, so they are an important part of a healthy daily diet. However, some include more sugar than others, especially dried fruits. You should aim to eat 2–3 portions of fruit per day, with one portion being what you can fit in your palm, but for dried fruits it should be 1 tablespoon (see page 34 for more on portion sizes).

ingredients on their packaging and many also list useful nutritional information, which can help you to see exactly what you are putting into your body. These labels include information on energy in kilojoules (kJ) and kilocalories (kcals), or calories, which is useful for those following a calorie-controlled diet.

The packet labels also include information about the amount of fat, saturated fat, carbohydrates, sugars, protein and salt. All nutritional information is provided per 100g and sometimes per portion of the food in each packet.

Some products will display a traffic light system for fat, saturated fat, sugars and salt: red means high, amber medium and green low. Anything that equates to high in these categories should be eaten in small amounts and in moderation.

What's high and what's low?

If you are not sure whether a food is high in saturated fat, sugar or salt, check the label, which will list guidelines such as:

TOTAL FAT
High: more than 17.5g (1 heaped tablespoon) of fat per 100g
Low: 3g (½ teaspoon) of fat or less per 100g

SATURATED FAT
High: more than 5g (1 teaspoon) of saturated fat per 100g
Low: 1.5g (less than ¼ teaspoon) of saturated fat or less per 100g

SUGARS
High: more than 22.5g (1½ tablespoons) of total sugars per 100g
Low: 5g (1 teaspoon) of total sugars or less per 100g

SALT
High: more than 1.5g (less than ¼ teaspoon) of salt per 100g (or 0.6g/pinch of sodium)
Low: 0.3g (pinch) of salt or less per 100g (or 0.1g/tiny pinch of sodium)

Each serving (150g) contains

Energy 1046kJ 250kcal	Fat 3.0g LOW	Saturates 1.3g LOW	Sugars 34g HIGH	Salt 0.9g MED
13%	4%	7%	38%	15%

of an adult's reference intake
Typical values (as sold) per 100g: 697kJ / 167kcal

Why eat more fruit and veg?

Fruit and vegetables are a good source of a variety of vitamins and minerals, including folate, vitamin C, potassium and phytonutrients (see box overleaf). They are also an excellent source of dietary fibre, which helps maintain a healthy gut (see page 38), prevents constipation and can also reduce the risk of bowel cancer. Most fruit and veg are low in fat and calories, too, which makes them a good choice for a healthy snack. Be warned, though, that dried fruits are higher in sugar (fructose) than fresh, and therefore calories, so these should be eaten in smaller quantities (see page 34, What is a portion?).

Try to fill half your plate at every meal with vegetables or salad ingredients. All fruit and vegetables contain different vitamins and minerals, so try to vary the types you eat for a range of flavours, textures and to get the optimum amount of vitamins. Don't forget that fruit and veg doesn't always have to be fresh; if you are on a budget or can't shop regularly, frozen, dried or tinned fruit are just as nutritious because they are packaged when freshly cropped, meaning fewer nutrients are lost. Check to see what liquid the fruit is tinned in, though – avoid fruit in syrups and opt for fresh juice to reduce the sugar content.

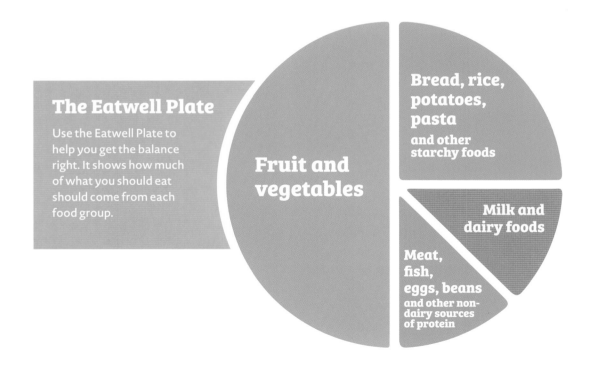

The Eatwell Plate

Use the Eatwell Plate to help you get the balance right. It shows how much of what you should eat should come from each food group.

Fruit and vegetables

Bread, rice, potatoes, pasta and other starchy foods

Milk and dairy foods

Meat, fish, eggs, beans and other non-dairy sources of protein

Eat the rainbow: phytonutrients

Phytonutrients – also known as phytochemicals – are natural compounds found in plant foods such as vegetables, fruit, wholegrain products and legumes, and are what gives fruit and vegetables their vibrant colours. Although not essential nutrients, they have beneficial effects in combination with other essential nutrients to promote good health, including antioxidant properties that help prevent damage to cells throughout the body. Some phytonutrients have been shown to reduce the risk of cancer, heart disease, stroke, Alzheimer's and Parkinson's disease.

Eating a rainbow of vegetables and fruit every day can help you to get many of the phytonutrients that nature has to offer and reduce the risk of illnesses, from the common cold to cancer. Good, phytonutrient-rich foods include:

- Red, orange and yellow vegetables and fruit (tomatoes, carrots, peppers, squash, sweet potatoes, peaches, mangos, melons, citrus fruits and berries)
- Dark green leafy vegetables (spinach, kale, broccoli, Swiss chard and romaine lettuce)
- Garlic, onions, chives and leeks
- Wholegrain products (brown and wild rice, quinoa, barley, wholewheat and wholegrain breads and wholegrain cereals)
- Nuts and seeds (walnuts, almonds, sunflower, sesame and flaxseeds)
- Legumes (dried beans, peas, lentils, soya beans and soya products)
- Tea and coffee (green, black and herbal teas)

Fats

Most diets are made up of different types of fats. Fats are often seen as the bad guys, in part because saturated fat is thought to be linked to high cholesterol levels (see page 48), which can cause coronary heart disease. However, not all are bad, so it is important to know what fats you are eating and to keep them in moderation – the Department of Health recommends that fats should not exceed 35% of our total daily energy (calorie) intake, and no more than 70g (about 4½ tablespoons) per day for adults.

Saturated fats

This is the fat that most adults eat too much of, and should be kept to minimum in a healthy daily diet. You will find these in butter and lard, fatty cuts of meat, sausages and bacon, processed foods such as pies, cakes and biscuits, and full-fat dairy products such as cheese and cream. The average man should have no more than 30g (2 tablespoons) of saturated fat per day, the average woman no more than 20g (1⅓ tablespoons) per day.

Wherever possible, replace saturated fats with small amounts of monounsaturated fats (these include olive oil, avocado, almonds and unsalted cashew nuts) or polyunsaturated fats (including sunflower and vegetable oils, sunflower seeds, walnuts and oily fish). These are a healthier choice and an important part of your diet because they provide essential fatty acids and fat-soluble vitamins (see page 24).

Trans fats

Trans fatty acids (also known as trans fats) are produced when vegetable oils are hydrogenated, which is a process that manufacturers use to prolong the shelf life and taste of their products. These are generally found in processed foods, and many major companies are under pressure to reduce the use of these, because they are linked to a rise in blood cholesterol and increasing levels of triglycerides – a form of blood fat. These impacts can raise your risk of coronary heart disease, so trans fats should be avoided wherever possible.

Omega 3

Western diets often tend to have a shortage of this polyunsaturated fat. Omega 3 is anti-inflammatory, helps prevent irregular heartbeats, helps ensure healthy blood clotting, reduces the build-up of fat in our arteries and plays an important part in helping to lower the level of LDL cholesterol in your blood (see page 48), all of which helps to keep your heart healthy. It is also thought to help inflammatory types of arthritis such as rheumatoid arthritis as it can reduce joint stiffness, and because it is beneficial for the brain, some studies have suggested that it could help to treat depression.

Good sources of omega 3 are flaxseeds, free-range eggs and oily fish, so it is recommended that we try to include oily fish such as salmon, mackerel, sardines, anchovies or herring in our diet once a week.

FACT
The National Diet and Nutrition Survey reveals Britons especially children aged 11 to 18 years get 14% of their daily calories from added sugar.

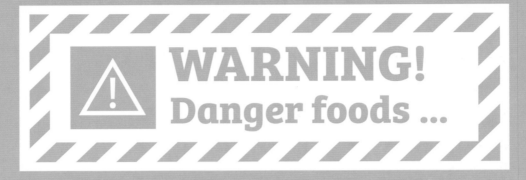

WARNING!
Danger foods ...

SUGAR – Sugary foods can really mess with our energy levels, raising them up and bringing them crashing back down, which can affect our mood and cause physical conditions such as tooth decay, weight gain, heart disease, certain cancers and Type 2 diabetes (see page 46).

Many foods contain natural sugars, such as fructose in fruit, and these foods also come packed with beneficial nutrients such as vitamins and fibre. The sugars to be wary of are the hidden refined sugars that are added to processed foods for flavouring or as preservatives. Look out for glucose, maltose, hydrolysed starch, molasses, corn syrup, sucrose, isoglucose and cane sugar on product labels for pasta sauces, fizzy drinks, flavoured water, squashes and cordials, alcohol, some breakfast cereals, dressings and condiments (ketchup and brown sauce), low-fat yoghurt and even bread. Some fruit juices can contain more sugar per 100ml than a can of cola – so always check the label!

We should only eat 30g (2 tablespoons) a day of added sugar – that's not much when you think that 1 tablespoon of ketchup contains 1 teaspoon of sugar, a 600ml sports drink contains the equivalent of 9½ teaspoons of sugar, and a large latte can contain 11 teaspoons.

SALT – Too much salt (or sodium) in the diet can cause raised blood pressure, which can increase your risk of heart disease and stroke. The total recommended daily allowance for salt is less than 6g (1 teaspoon) for adults, half that for children up to 6 years old, so you should try to reduce the amount of salt you consume as much as possible – both within the foods you buy or cook and, more importantly, by avoiding adding salt to cooked food. This doesn't mean eating bland foods – you can add flavour with herbs and spices instead, and you can retrain your palate to enjoy these subtler flavours. As with sugar, there can be hidden salt in some foods, such as in breakfast cereals, dressings and condiments, bread, sausages, ham and salamis, smoked meat and fish, cheese, ready meals, crisps and bought pizza and pasta sauces and salted or dry roasted nuts.

FACT
Britain is overdosing on salt, consuming on average 8.6g per day – 43% more than the recommendation – and this is responsible for between 14–20,000 deaths from cardiovascular disease each year.

Protein

Protein is an essential nutrient – one of the three main food groups – which is needed by the body for cell growth and repair, including building tissue and muscles. The building blocks of protein are amino acids, and different foods contain different amounts and combinations of these amino acids. Protein from animal sources (meat, fish, eggs and dairy products) contains the full range of 20 essential amino acids needed by the body; however, to get all the amino acids they need, vegans and vegetarians should combine different plant sources of protein, such as pulses, peas and cereals to get a complete protein intake (the Vegetarian Society – vegsoc.org – has more information for combining food groups to get a complete protein count). The recommended daily allowance for protein is 50g (just over 3 tablespoons) for adults.

Meat – good or bad?

Some people choose not to eat meat for reasons of taste, ethics about animal rearing or the impact on the environment. Scientists believe we should be aiming to reduce our meat and dairy intake by 70% in order to protect the planet. Methane emissions from cows and the land and water climate footprint connected to rearing meat, which can be 10–100 times greater than that of cultivating plant-based foods. Reducing our intake by 70 per cent translates as eating one portion each of chicken and fish per week and red meat once a month.

The recommended daily intake of meat is between 70 and 90g of lean cuts of red meat, as it is a really nutritious food – full of vitamins, minerals and a source of complete proteins, but if you eat processed meat or too much red meat you can increase your risk of developing cardiovascular disease, Type 2 diabetes and certain cancers like bowel cancer. So the answer is to strike a balance for your health and that of the planet, and also to consider buying organic or sustainably reared meat and dairy products, which you know will have been produced with consideration of environmental issues.

Fibre

It is important to get enough fibre (also known as roughage) into our diets for a number of reasons, including supporting healthy bowel function and reducing the risk of constipation, and helping to balance blood-sugar and energy levels. Research has also shown that a fibre-rich diet can help increase the good bacteria in the gut (see page 39) and reduce your risk of bowel cancer, heart disease and stroke, and Type 2 diabetes. The recommended daily allowance for fibre is 30g (2 tablespoons) per day for adults – a small handful of unsalted nuts can include 3g of fibre, two slices of wholemeal bread provides 6.5g, one medium apple around 13.6g, and a small glass of fresh smoothie around 9.4g.

The European Food Safety Authority has also suggested that fibre-rich foods can help you to lose and maintain a healthy weight.

Good fibre-rich foods include:
- Wholegrain breakfast cereals and bread, oats, wholewheat pasta, barley and rye
- Fruit – in particular oranges, lemons, berries, pears and melon
- Vegetables such as broccoli, carrots and sweetcorn, and potatoes with skin left on
- Peas, beans and pulses
- Nuts and seeds

Vitamins

You can get all the vitamins you need from a balanced and varied diet, without the need for buying expensive supplements. Vitamins are nutrients required by the body in small amounts, for a variety of essential processes, and as most vitamins cannot be made by the body, they must be provided through diet.

There are two types of vitamins – **fat-soluble** and **water-soluble**.

Fat-soluble vitamins

These vitamins are mainly found in foods that are high in natural fats such as animal fats, vegetable oils, dairy foods, liver and oily fish. These include vitamins A, D, E and K. Your body needs these vitamins to work properly, but it is efficient at storing them, so you don't need to eat foods containing them every day.

Vitamin A: Helps your immune system to fight infections, improves vision in dim light and keeps skin and hair healthy.

Found in: Meat, eggs, dairy and oily fish as beta-carotene (which our bodies convert to vitamin A), fruit and vegetables such as broccoli, dark green leafy veg, sweet potatoes, red peppers, squash, mangoes and apricots. The recommended daily allowance for vitamin A is 700µg for men, 600µg for women.

Vitamin D: Helps to regulate the amount of calcium and phosphate in the body, which is important for bone, teeth and muscle health. It is also believed to help prevent some cancers and works with vitamins A and C to support the immune system. Vitamin D can be made by the body in the skin when it is exposed to sunlight, which is another good reason to get outside and into the sunshine regularly for at least 15–30 minutes each day between late March and September – housebound people often need to take a supplement for good health.

Found in: Salmon, herring and mackerel, red meat and offal – liver and kidney – egg yolks and fortified cereals, soya products and spreads. The recommended daily allowance for vitamin D is 10µg for adults.

Vitamin E: An antioxidant that's needed to repair damaged cells and for healthy skin and a well-functioning immune system.

Found in: All vegetable oils, such as sunflower and pumpkin oils, as well as tuna, salmon, broccoli, almonds, eggs, soya and wholegrains, which include oats, rye and brown rice. The recommended daily allowance for vitamin A is 4µg for men, 3µg for women.

Vitamin K: Important for healthy bones and blood clotting, an essential part of healing.

Found in: Yoghurt, egg yolks, fish oils, dairy produce and green leafy vegetables. The recommended daily allowance for vitamin K is 1µg per kilogram of body weight.

Water-soluble vitamins

Unlike fat-soluble vitamins, these vitamins aren't stored in the body and any excess that the body doesn't use is expelled through your urine, so you need to make sure you eat foods with these vitamins regularly. Water-soluble vitamins include vitamin C, the B vitamins and folic acid.

Vitamin B1: Also known as thiamin, B1 is needed for energy production, digesting carbohydrates, a healthy nervous system and heart function.

Found in: Wholegrain foods such as cereals and bread, oats, rye millet, quinoa, legumes, pork and liver. The recommended daily allowance for vitamin B1 is 1µg for men, 0.8µg for women.

Vitamin B2: Also known as riboflavin, vitamin B2 helps to keep the skin, eyes and nervous system healthy and works to release energy from the food you eat.

Found in: Milk, eggs, fortified breakfast cereals and rice. Vitamin B2 is destroyed by UV light so keep foods out of sunlight. The recommended daily allowance for vitamin B2 is 1.3µg for men, 1.1µg for women.

Vitamin B3: Also called niacin, vitamin B3 is good for hormone synthesis, such as insulin (which regulates blood sugar levels in the body), thyroxine, serotonin and other mood and brain hormones, so it is thought to be useful for conditions including depression, arthritis and circulatory disorders.

Found in: High-protein foods such as chicken, beef, fish and nuts. Breads and cereals are often enriched with niacin. The recommended daily allowance for vitamin B3 is 16.5µg for men, 13.2µg for women.

Vitamin B5: Also known as pantothenic acid, this is needed for the conversion of fats and carbohydrates into energy and for supporting the adrenal glands, which regulate the stress response in the body.

Found in: Fish, poultry, wholegrains, rye, barley, millet, nuts, chicken, egg yolks, liver and green leafy vegetables. No recommended daily allowance is set for this vitamin.

Vitamin B6: Involved in more bodily processes than any other vitamin, vitamin B6 forms red blood cells, helps cells to make proteins and manufactures neurotransmitters in the brain.

Found in: Poultry, lean red meat, egg yolks, chickpeas, oily fish, cabbage, leeks, bananas, all dairy produce and wheatgerm. The recommended daily allowance for vitamin B6 is 1.4µg for men, 1.2µg for women.

Vitamin B9: Better known as folic acid, vitamin B9 is known for its role in helping to prevent neural defects during pregnancy but it is also good for the immune system, energy production and in preventing anaemia.

Found in: Dark green leafy vegetables such as kale, spinach, asparagus, broccoli, sprouts, egg yolks, carrots, apricots, oranges, pumpkins and squashes, melons, wholewheat and rye. The recommended daily allowance for folic acid is 200µg for adults, 400µg for women trying for a baby or until they are 12 weeks pregnant.

Vitamin B12: Needed for growth, the digestive and nervous system, as well as the production of energy and healthy blood cells. After the age of 50, the ability to absorb vitamin B12 from food declines.

Found in: Animal products, including red meat – beef, liver and pork, shellfish and fish, eggs and dairy produce. Vegetarians can get B12 from seaweed and spirulina. The recommended daily allowance for vitamin B12 is 1.5µg for adults.

Vitamin C: Also known as ascorbic acid, vitamin C helps to support the immune system, a healthy heart, skin and gums, and to prevent diseases like heart disease and cancer and to help wounds to heal properly.

Found in: Berries, pomegranates, citrus fruits, potatoes, pumpkins, cabbage, broccoli, cauliflower and spinach. The recommended daily allowance for vitamin C is 40µg for adults.

Minerals

Your body needs certain minerals to build strong bones and teeth and turn the food you eat into energy. Just as with vitamins, a healthy balanced diet should provide all the minerals your body needs.

There are many minerals, but the essential ones you need to make sure that you are getting are calcium, iron and potassium.

Calcium: An important component in the activity of many enzymes in the body and is essential for building and maintaining bones and teeth. In periods of growth, and during pregnancy and breastfeeding you may need more calcium.

Found in: Dairy produce, small-boned fish such as sardines and anchovies, green leafy vegetables, nuts and seeds such as almonds and sesame seeds, tofu and apricots. The recommended daily allowance for calcium is 700µg for adults.

Iron: A critical mineral, iron is vital for the production of red blood cells, transporting oxygen from the lungs to the body's tissues and taking carbon dioxide from the tissues to the lungs. Iron functions in several key enzymes in energy production and metabolism. Iron deficiency can cause anaemia, which is very common, particularly in menstruating women and teenage girls.

Found in: Red meat, sardines, offal, egg yolks and fortified cereals. Your body better absorbs iron if it is taken with vitamin C, so drink fruit juice or eat fruit and veg with your iron-rich meal. Tea, on the other hand, interferes with iron absorption, so wait for about an hour before drinking it. The recommended daily allowance for iron is 8.7µg for men, 14.8µg for women aged 19 to 50, and 8.7µg for women over 50.

Keeping hydrated

Water is an essential ingredient in our diet because our bodies are 50–75 per cent water, so drinking enough liquids to keep the fluid levels in the body topped up helps to ensure that all vital bodily functions can occur.

Water in the body is essential for our blood system to carry essential glucose, oxygen and nutrients to cells, to help the kidneys get rid of waste products, and it also lubricates our joints and eyes, helps our digestive system to function optimally and keeps our skin healthy. It is also, of course, vital in helping us to regulate our body temperature through perspiration, so in hot weather or after physical activity it is important to replace any fluids that are lost to prevent dehydration. Dehydration – which is caused when we have low levels of fluid in the body – can cause headaches, dizziness, lethargy, poor concentration and a dry mouth. Over a longer period, dehydration can cause constipation and can be linked with urinary tract infections and kidney stones.

Another good reason for drinking water is that sometimes you might think you are hungry but in fact you are thirsty; when you drink, you suppress your appetite and therefore the temptation to overeat. Regular hydration has been shown to help weight loss and maintenance, and if you are drinking water, it is 100 per cent calorie-free.

How much do I need?

Adults and teenagers need to drink around 1.5–2 litres of fluid a day; children need slightly less and should aim for 1–1.5 litres a day. If you are not sure if you are drinking enough, a good indicator is urine colour – pale straw-coloured urine tells you that you have good hydration levels, while darker-coloured urine is a sign that the body needs more fluid.

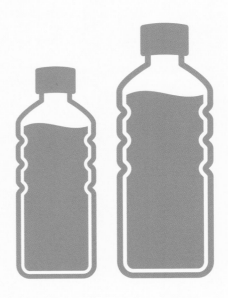

Which drinks count?

Any drink will help you to stay hydrated. Water is the best option, though, because it contains no other additives, such as sugars and fats, but milk, fruit juice, tea, coffee and soft drinks can all help to top up fluid levels. Homemade smoothies made from blended fruits and vegetables will not only hydrate but also have the added bonus of all the nutrients that come from these foods. Be careful not to have drinks with higher levels of added sugars, such as fizzy drinks and cordials, and even some fruit juices; these will not only cause dental problems but also an increased risk of developing Type 2 diabetes. Drinks with added cream or full-fat milk also provide more calories, so make drinks like creamy hot chocolates or lattes a treat.

Tips for staying hydrated

- Start the day as you mean to go on – drink a glass of water first thing, or a mug of hot water and lemon juice.

- Buy yourself a water bottle and keep it with you to remind yourself to keep drinking – pop it on your desk, take it out with you whenever you go out. Top it up throughout the day.

- Don't wait until you're thirsty to drink. If you are feeling thirsty, you are already becoming dehydrated. Drink little and often throughout the day.

- If you find water boring, perk it up with a slice of fresh fruit or some fruit-filled ice cubes to add a bit of natural flavour without added sugar.

- Eat water-rich foods – some juicy fruits and vegetables are over 90% water; try courgettes, cucumber, tomatoes, watermelon or cantaloupe melon, strawberries and peaches.

- If it's a really hot day, wear loose-fitting clothes and stay out of the sun to reduce water loss through perspiration.

TIME TO GET COOKING!

We all have busy lives, and we all know how tempting it is to reach for a ready meal or a takeaway menu after a long day. But these foods are often high in saturated and trans fats, sugar, salt and all sorts of artificial additives, so while they might fill a hunger gap, they won't be feeding your body with all that it needs.

Preparing your own food means you are in complete control of what you are putting into your body, which is vital if you are sticking to a specific diet – whether to manage weight loss, an allergy, boost your mood or for other health reasons. One of the best reasons to cook your own food from scratch is the fact that you can use really fresh and nutritious ingredients and it gives you the opportunity to include healthy flavourings, such as natural herbs and spices, rather than salt, artificial additives and sugar.

Cooking from scratch can also be significantly cheaper, as the raw products will be much less expensive than pre-prepared food or takeaways. Preparing your own food also means you could get into the habit of taking breakfast or lunch to work with you, either specially prepared or using last night's leftovers; a working couple could each spend £40 a week on takeaway lunches, coffee and snacks, which works out at an eyewatering £4000 a year between them! If you need an incentive to avoid picking up food from a shop on the way to work, keep a jar handy and pop the money you've saved into it ready to buy yourself a treat – not necessarily a food-based one!

Planning ahead

As we discussed earlier, planning your meals will make your time spent in the kitchen much easier and less stressful. Choose recipes that are popular with your household and that everyone will eat – either ones you know or some from pages 62–207 in this book. Try to rotate them, and maybe pick a few new ones to cook each week so that you get a bit of variety and interest in your diet.

Deciding on recipes in advance saves you staring into a fridge for inspiration after a long day, and it makes shopping easier and cheaper, too, because you will have everything to hand, and you only buy the food that you need, so there should be less wastage. Don't try to be ambitious on busy week nights, be realistic about how much time you have to cook – if it becomes a chore or complicated you'll be back reaching for the ready meals. If you're new to cooking, start with the basics and build your skills as you grow in confidence.

Think about what you and your family like and dislike when you are choosing what to eat, and consider any dietary requirements – such as allergies – and this will make it much easier to stick to the plan. If you know you have a busy evening one day of the week, plan something really quick and easy to prepare, or even think about a one-pot meal that family members can reheat if they are getting home at different times.

Aaagh! I've never cooked in my life!

If you're new to cooking and feeling a bit nervous or overwhelmed at the idea, here are a few tips to get you started.

- Read the recipe before you start and get everything you need in front of you. If you are missing an ingredient, don't panic, you might be able to easily substitute with something you do have, or just leave it out.

- Defrost any frozen ingredients in advance – particularly meat, chicken or fish. Vegetables will defrost quickly when cooked, so it's perfectly okay to chuck in some frozen veg.

- Preheat the oven when the recipe tells you to, so that the oven is nice and hot when you need it. Grease and line any tins at the start, too.

- Check the cooking instructions on any packets, such as pasta or rice.

- Clear up as you go, then you won't have the depressing sight of a kitchen full of pans when you've eaten and just want to relax. Get all the other members of your household involved with this!

Find your favourites

Keep a note of recipes that worked well for you, time-wise, but also that were popular with you or the family. Having a batch of go-to recipes will help keep you kitchen confident and engaged with cooking at home.

Batch-cooking can also provide you with delicious homemade meals that you can pull out of the fridge or freezer when you're short of time or ingredients (see page 35).

Take into account food for breakfasts, lunch, dinner and snacks, and any packed lunches you might need. (See page 210 for a template meal planner.) When you have your shopping list, whether you're shopping online or in-store, don't get sidetracked by tempting offers or treats – stick to the list and you'll keep to your budget and your health goals. When you're in the supermarket, think fresh and wholefood. Choose good protein sources, such as eggs, fish, healthy cuts of meat, and focus on wholegrains, fruit and veg. Think variety, choose a range of ingredients for flavour, colour and texture.

Clever tricks for meeting your fruit and veg targets!

If you are struggling to think of how to get more fruit and veg into your daily diet, try some of these ideas.

BREAKFAST:

Add fresh, frozen or tinned fruit, sliced apple, banana or fresh berries to pancakes, a dollop of natural yoghurt, or some porridge. Blend fruit into smoothies, or mash bananas or fresh strawberries and whisk them into milk for a healthy and low-sugar milkshake.

Make your own granola (see page 70) with your favourite dried fruits.

If you like a cooked breakfast, make the plate mostly veg – grill mushrooms or tomatoes, cook some spinach to serve alongside scrambled eggs or bacon.

LUNCH:

Put together a salad (see pages 100–132), pack a sandwich or a wholemeal tortilla with lettuce, tomatoes, cucumber, peppers or grated carrot or chop up some raw veg to eat with a low-fat dip or hummus. Cook up some veg and beans to eat as a soup.

DINNER:

Fill half your plate with veg! Add tinned, frozen or chopped vegetables such as carrots, peas or mushrooms to soups, stews, Bolognese sauce or homemade burgers.

Cook up a stir-fry – eat the rainbow! Pack in peppers, onion, broccoli, beansprouts, carrots and any stray vegetables in your fridge.

If you need a sweet fix, make a fresh fruit salad, and, if you like, serve with yoghurt, or try the fruit dishes in the sweet treats section. Any leftovers can always be eaten for breakfast.

Storecupboard staples

If your planning has gone awry, or your shopping is missing some vital ingredients, it's a good idea to have your kitchen well-stocked with a few essentials. Often tinned or dried, these ingredients tend to have a long shelf life and provide a useful base for many recipes.

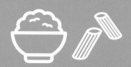

RICE, PASTA, GRAINS AND PULSES

Wholegrain or wild rice, for use in salads, sides and risottos; a selection of dried pasta shapes, for sauces, salads and in soups; dried noodles (egg or rice) for stir-fries; couscous and pearl barley for veggie tagines or stews, salads and soups; pulses and beans, for salads and stews.

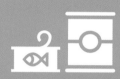

TINS

Any vegetables, especially tomatoes for sauces.

Fish – tuna, salmon, sardines or anchovies for pasta sauces or salads.

Fruit – peaches, pineapple, cherries, mandarin, etc. to add to yoghurt, or top with granola for a speedy crumble.

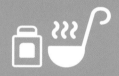

SEASONINGS FOR ADDING FLAVOUR

Dried herbs and spices such as oregano, smoked paprika, chilli, cinnamon, cumin, coriander, curry powder or paste, five-spice, turmeric, ginger, fennel seeds, sea salt and pepper.

Low-salt stock cubes.

OILS AND VINEGARS

Vegetable oil and olive oil. Red wine, white wine, cider and balsamic vinegars for marinades, dressings and sauces.

BAKING STAPLES AND EXTRAS

Plain flour, self-raising flour and baking powder. Bread flour and dried yeast for making bread and pizza dough.

Cocoa powder and vanilla extract for flavouring. Caster, granulated and icing sugars.

Porridge oats – for porridge, granola, cookies, flapjacks and crumbles.

Nuts and seeds – for toasting and sprinkling over salads, or eating as a healthy snack.

Portion sizes – how much is enough?

Healthy eating is all about eating well, but not overeating. One of the biggest causes of obesity is super-sized portions, and reducing the amount we serve up will have a big impact on our waistlines and our general health – not to mention our wallets! Eating just 100kcals a day above the recommended daily allowance will mean that by the end of a year you will have gained an extra 10lbs in weight.

Studies have shown that if you put too much on your plate you will most likely eat it all, because so many of us were told as children to eat everything up. So reduce the temptation to eat more than you actually need and scale back your portion sizes.

If you're not used to cooking or you are not following a recipe and just preparing a meal off the cuff, it's really easy to make

What is a portion?

A single portion per food group that you are putting on your plate should weigh about 80g (just over 5 tablespoons) for adults, which is roughly equivalent to:

3 tablespoons cooked vegetables

A small bowl of salad

1 apple, orange, banana or pear

1 large slice of melon or pineapple

2 plums, kiwi fruit or satsumas

1 glass of pure fruit juice (including from concentrate)

1 tablespoon dried fruit

3 sticks of celery, 1 medium raw carrot or 5-cm piece of cucumber, or 7 cherry tomatoes

For children, a portion is as much as they can hold in their hand.

too much. So, always weigh out food according to the recipe, and get into the habit of weighing out pasta or rice (one recommended portion is 80g uncooked pasta/rice/noodles – about the size of your fist). Don't forget, weighing out food is an economical way of cooking, too, as it reduces food waste.

Keep those portion sizes down!

- Don't starve yourself between meals, because if you do you will be more likely to overeat. Eat one or two healthy snacks during the day, such as a piece of fruit or raw veg. This will keep hunger pangs at bay.

- Drinking a glass of water before eating will fill you up so you eat less.

- Use smaller plates such as side plates instead of dinner plates, or make sure you keep a decent border clear around the edge of your plate.

- If you think your plate looks a bit empty, fill the gaps with vegetables or salad.

- Eat slowly and mindfully – focus on your food, don't eat while working, reading, watching TV or scrolling through your phone. If you are aware of how much you are eating, you will also be aware of when you are feeling full. Ask yourself, am I still hungry?

Cooking for busy days

Batch-cooking is a brilliant way to get ahead for busy days, by putting pre-cooked homemade food in the freezer ready to pull out whenever you need it. It's also a great way to save money, as you can take advantage of food offers in supermarkets such as buy one get one free, or marked-down ingredients that need to be cooked quickly, or to use up any leftovers or ingredients in the fridge so you don't waste them.

If you've never done it before, this might sound time-consuming, but in fact it only takes the same amount of time as preparing one meal – you're just cooking double the quantity. It can also be a great way to spend a slow afternoon; you could cook a few different meals to go into the fridge or freezer for the week or weeks ahead, either storing them in bulk or in individual portions. If you don't have time to prepare a complete meal, you could just make the base of a meal – a pasta sauce or pizza base, or some fresh stock.

It is time well spent; having homemade food to hand will keep you on track with healthy eating, because on those nights when you're too tired to cook it will reduce the temptation to reach for a shop-bought ready meal.

Get organised before you start batch cooking:

- Create the space – clear out the freezer so it is ready to store your pre-prepared dinners. Have an 'eat from the freezer' day or two and sort out any outdated food to free up some space.

- Buy a load of cheap freezerproof containers with lids to store your meals in – foil ones are good if you want to transfer the dishes straight from freezer to the oven when you need them (or use microwave-proof containers if you prefer).

- Clearly label any food you store and add the date of freezing – food can be frozen for 3–6 months.

- If you can, try to divide whatever you are storing in the freezer into portions, so that nothing gets wasted when you defrost it, as you can't refreeze it.

Time-saving gadgets

If you want to eat healthily but you really don't want to spend your free time in the kitchen standing over the hob, slow cookers and pressure cookers are fantastic for taking over the cooking for you.

Slow cookers are great for leaving food cooking while you get on with something else, and are ideal for batch cooking. They cook gradually, over 6–8 hours, but use much less electricity than a standard oven, and can be left on during the day or overnight.

If you want dinner quickly, **pressure cookers** will cook your food in half the time stated in most recipes. Slow cookers and pressure cookers are really good at preserving nutrients in food, because they are one-pot machines, so nutrients are not lost into the cooking water and then drained away.

If you have space, a **food processor** makes light work of blending, making crumbs, grating and chopping, and making pastry. **Mini blenders** and **hand-held electric blenders** are useful for blending smoothies, soups, pestos, sauces and even hard ingredients.

Love your leftovers

Hopefully you'll soon be really efficient at managing your food portions so you won't have any leftovers, but if you do, don't be tempted to go back for seconds. Instead, save them for another day or another meal. Pasta or rice can be used as the base for a cold salad, vegetables can be blended into soups, chicken or meat can be eaten in sandwiches or used in stir-fries, risottos, pasta sauces or soups.

Before you go and do your weekly shop, have a rummage through your fridge – unused veg, cheese and meats, chicken or fish can be cooked up and frozen to save waste. For example, roast old bits of veg and store as ratatouille, grate odd bits of lefotver cheese and freeze as it is or use it to make cheese sauce, whizz stale bread in a food processor to make breadcrumbs that you can use in recipes later.

If you are keeping leftovers from cooked food, cool them at room temperature, ideally within 1–2 hours, cover, then transfer to the fridge immediately, where they can be stored for up to 2 days. If you have a large amount, spread the food out into a large, shallow dish so it cools quicker. If your cooked leftovers haven't previously been frozen, you can also put them in the freezer, if you prefer.

When you come to reheat, defrost frozen food at room temperature, and then cook it gently, making sure the food is heated all the way through until piping hot. Don't reheat leftovers more than once.

Tips on freezing

- Some foods don't survive the freezing process well, losing their texture once defrosted. These include vegetables with a high water content, such as lettuce, cucumber, radishes and mushrooms and ingredients with a higher fat content, such as cream, egg-based sauces, yoghurt and low-fat soft cheese.
- Only freeze foods once they are completely cold.
- Don't freeze foods that have previously been frozen.
- Store foods in portions to save wastage on defrosting and always label with the contents and date of freezing.
- In general, freeze homemade foods for up to 3 months.

GUT HEALTH

The gut is finally getting all the praise and attention it deserves. This hugely underrated workhorse of our bodies has been the subject of increased research, as numerous studies have linked gut health to the immune system, mood, mental health, autoimmune diseases, endocrine disorders, skin conditions, cancer, heart disease, liver disease, diabetes, asthma, depression, autism, irritable bowel syndrome, Parkinson's and many allergies.

Your gut microbiome weighs about 2kg and is bigger than the human brain. For every person it is a busy community that contains between 300 and 500 different species of bacteria, and it is located in your intestine. The microbiome that make up this community provide us with an unbelievable array of different functions that keep us and our gut healthy. This includes programming our immune system, helping to digest the food that we eat, fighting off nasty bacteria and playing a critical role in weight regulation.

The microbes that live in our gut – and in our poo – digest the food that we eat. What you eat can have an effect on the performance of your microbes, so it is important to think about what you're putting into your gut ecosystem to be able to give your good gut bacteria the support they need to do their work. To keep the gut microbiome healthy, we need to think about feeding it moisture and nutrients. If we don't provide it with the right quantities or the right types, this ecosystem in our gut can start to grow or become damaged, which will negatively impact our health.

Gut feeling

Have you ever felt that your gut is reflecting your mood? Well, it's true, our gut holds up to 90% of the body's serotonin, the neurotransmitter (aka chemical messenger) that is responsible for mood, and there is evidence in continuing studies that a healthy gut (microbiome) can improve certain cognitive processes and mood. This is because the gut has its own nervous system, the enteric nervous system, which contains 100 million neurons. The gut-brain axis is a two-way street, which shoots neurotransmitters produced within the gut around the body and to the brain via the vagus nerve.

Gut bacteria and your poo

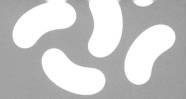

Poo is a subject that isn't standard chat for most people, unsurprisingly, but it is a hugely important source of information for scientists. Your poo contains trillions and trillions of microbes, which reveal a whole host of different beneficial functions that keep us healthy every day. So for scientists, poo presents a snapshot of what's happening inside our gut and is a rich resource for study; they are able to look inside it and see what microbes are there. They can also identify which special molecules or compounds these microbes might be producing in order to better understand why they are really important for our health and wellbeing.

Your poo changes, even from day to day, and this can give a window into your overall health and gut health – for example, analysis of the bacteria in our gut can predict obesity in the person it has come from with an accuracy of 90%. It will also reveal to you if you are eating enough fibre and if you are hydrated enough.

If you want to check out if your poo is healthy, have a look at the Bristol Stool Chart below and compare the consistency of it – the pictures can show you how healthy a poo is on a scale of one to seven. One and two might mean you are potentially constipated, three or four is the ideal poo that you want to be producing each day.

The Bristol Stool Chart

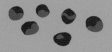

Type 1
Separate hard lumps, like nuts (hard to pass)

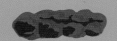

Type 2
Sausage-shaped but lumpy

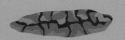

Type 3
Like a sausage but with a cracked surface

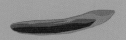

Type 4
Like a sausage or snake, smooth and soft

Type 5
Soft blobs with clear-cut edges (passed easily)

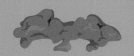

Type 6
Fluffy pieces with ragged edges, quite mushy

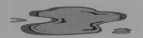

Type 7
No solid pieces – entirely liquid

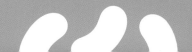

Eating right for your microbes

What you eat isn't just nutrition for you, it also feeds the trillions of bacteria that live in your gut, so if you want to improve your digestion, lose weight or just look after your general health, there are some food guidelines you should follow:

- Eat a wide range of plant-based foods. A healthy gut has a diverse community of microbes, each of which prefers different foods.

- Eat more fibre (see page 24), aiming for at least the recommended daily intake of 2 tablespoons. Most people eat less than they should. Some people find cereals and grains can cause bloating and irritable bowel syndrome. If that's the case for you, get your fibre from fruit and vegetables instead.

- Drink plenty of fluids. Fibre acts like a sponge, absorbing water, so your gut needs fluids to help it to move waste through your digestive system and to soften poo and prevent constipation. Water is the best and healthiest option,

but if you prefer variety, choose drinks that are not fizzy and do not contain caffeine, such as herbal teas and milk.

- Avoid highly processed foods, which often contain ingredients that either suppress 'good' bacteria or increase 'bad' bacteria.

- Greasy and fatty foods, such as chips, burgers and fried foods, are also harder to digest and can cause stomach pain and heartburn. Try to eat more lean meat and fish, drink skimmed or semi-skimmed milk, and grill rather than fry foods.

- Go easy on spice. Although many people can eat spicy food with no ill-effects on their digestive system, others can find it upsets their gut, and that includes onion and garlic as well as hot ingredients like chillies.

- Include gut-friendly probiotics and prebiotics in your diet.

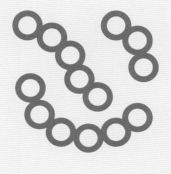

Gut-friendly bacteria

There is a lot of talk about prebiotics and probiotics, but do they genuinely help our gut health?

Probiotics – the so-called 'friendly bacteria' – are healthy bacteria, while the job of prebiotics is to feed these healthy bacteria. By including prebiotics in our diet, we can help our gut bacteria to grow strong so that they can keep our overall ecosystem working optimally. Probiotics have been linked to all sorts of digestive health benefits, including helping irritable bowel syndrome and diarrhoea.

Probiotics are found naturally in the gut and in fermented foods and live yoghurt, or you can take them as supplements. Prebiotics come from plant-based foods such as artichokes, asparagus, bananas, berries, tomatoes, garlic, onions, legumes, green vegetables and wholegrain cereals, so you should be able to get probiotics and prebiotics from a healthy balanced diet.

Other foods that are being researched as potentially good for the gut include:

- Fermented foods, such as sauerkraut, kimchi, miso, kombucha and many pickles. These are rich in probiotic bacteria and are easier to digest than a lot of foods because some of the sugars and starches within them have already been broken down during the process of fermentation. These foods are cheap and easy to make yourself and it's better to do so, as mass-produced pickles use vinegar instead of traditional methods of fermentation, so they don't have the same benefits as homemade versions.

Antibiotics and your gut

Antibiotics can be really important for fighting infections, but try not to take them unless it's completely necessary. This is because antibiotics cannot discriminate between the good bacteria and the bad ones, which means that a course of antibiotics might kill off some of your beneficial bacteria, too. If you really need to take antibiotics, make sure you eat lots of foods that boost your microbes afterwards.

- Sourdough bread is made by slow fermentation, using a wide range of bacteria and fungi found naturally in the air and in the ingredients used to make them. Many people claim they find sourdough easier to digest than other bread. However, this could be because the lengthy fermentation process is beneficial as the microbes have had more time to break down the protein strands that can cause digestive problems.

- Cheese produced by traditional methods that use natural bacteria can contain a huge array of probiotics. Some studies have found that these can benefit health, but more research is required.

- Traditionally produced yoghurts, 'live' yoghurts and yoghurt drinks contain probiotic cultures, but we don't know if they survive the acidic environment of the stomach and go on to reach the intestines intact.

Beware of triggering foods

If you find that you are regularly experiencing digestive issues after eating, keep a food diary and try to identify which foods are causing the problem, then begin to exclude them and see if symptoms improve.

There are some particular foods that have a reputation for irritating the gut.

- Acidic foods, such as tomatoes, citrus fruits, salad dressings, and drinks with caffeine (such as coffee, colas, tea and some fizzy drinks), boost acid in the stomach, which can trigger heartburn. Wheat and onions may cause irritable bowel syndrome.

- If you find you are developing wind and diarrhoea after drinking milk or eating dairy products, including cream, cheese, yoghurt and chocolate, it could be that you are struggling to digest lactose, the sugar that is in milk. See your doctor to test for an allergy or intolerance.

- If you already have a problem like heartburn or an irritable bowel, avoid spicy foods completely.

EATING FOR SPECIFIC HEALTH ISSUES

Healthy eating isn't just about keeping to a healthy weight or eating a balanced diet to keep your body functioning optimally, it can also alleviate or help reduce the risk of contracting the symptoms of numerous illnesses and health conditions.

Mood food – eating for optimal mental health

It's true, what you eat can affect you mentally as well as physically. There is evidence that suggests that what you eat can improve your mood (see page 38), give you more energy and prevent brain fog so you can think more clearly. Similarly, improving your mental health can help you escape the pattern of eating high-sugar foods when you're feeling emotional or to boost your mood or energy. Eating patterns like these lead to obesity or eating disorders in an attempt to prevent weight gain.

To 'declutter' your mind and brain, you need to focus on eating well, but it also helps to do this in combination with taking adequate exercise (too much is as bad as too little), managing your stress levels, getting sufficient sleep and getting sufficient daily sun exposure to boost your vitamin D (see page 25).

The relationship between diet and mental health is complex, but there is evidence that some foods can boost our mood. Following a Mediterranean-style diet (one with lots of vegetables, seafood, fresh herbs, garlic, olive oil, cereal and grains) and a range of fermented foods to keep gut microbes happy has been found in some studies to reduce the symptoms of depression. There is also some research to show that small amounts of grass-fed, high-quality red meat can reduce our risk of mental health problems. This is because it is much higher in the omega 3s, linked to improved mental health compared to the meat of grain-fed beef. Again, to maintain a healthy balanced diet and do our bit for the environment, we should try to eat high-quality meat in small amounts, bulking out dishes with beans, pulses and vegetables.

Some foods can prevent the conversion of others into nutrients that we need to support correct brain function. These include saturated fats, butter, lard and palm oil. Other foods can have a negative effect on the brain, tricking it into releasing mood-changing chemicals. These include caffeine, chocolate and sugary snacks. Caffeine is a stimulant, so it will perk you up quickly, but it might leave you feeling anxious and can disrupt your sleep if it is drunk after 4pm. Sugary foods will also give you a rapid energy boost, but as your sugar levels drop you will be left feeling tired, irritable and depressed.

Your gut can also feel the effects of your emotions, and if you are feeling stressed or anxious your gut activity can speed up or slow down. Including lots of fibre in your diet and other gut-friendly foods (see page 41) and staying hydrated will help to regulate this.

Feed your mood

FOODS TO AVOID:

High-sugar foods, such as sweets, biscuits, cakes

Fats in fried food, trans fats, fats in processed meats

Sugary drinks

Caffeine

Alcohol

FOODS TO INCLUDE:

Slow-release foods: pasta, rice, oats, wholegrain bread and cereals and nuts and seeds.

Salmon, mackerel, tuna and other fatty fish

Blueberries

Spinach and other leafy greens

Yoghurt and other probiotic foods (see page 41)

Dark chocolate

Hormones – diet and the menopause

The menopause is a time of raging hormones and change, and every woman will experience symptoms to varying degrees of severity. Some women can be perimenopausal three to fifteen years before they actually enter the menopause (the average age in the UK is 51 for the menopause), so it is a good idea to get into beneficial eating habits well in advance.

The production of oestrogen and progesterone from the ovaries starts to decline from the age of 35 as egg reserves start to run out. Progesterone declines more rapidly than oestrogen, which can tip you into oestrogen dominance. Oestrogen levels can fluctuate wildly during perimenopause, so you can experience a range of symptoms, such as hot flushes, night sweats, difficulty in sleeping, headaches, low mood, anxiety and decreased libido. Not all women experience all these symptoms, but for most women it can still be an emotional rollercoaster as your body tries to compensate for the decline of oestrogen.

For severe symptoms, the doctor might prescribe hormone replacement therapy, but there are other things you can do to manage the symptoms of the menopause, including reducing your stress levels, avoiding triggers such as caffeine, smoking and alcohol – and eating a healthy diet.

Foods for the menopause

Good digestion is really important because it helps eliminate excess oestrogen, so make sure your diet includes 30g fibre daily (see page 24). Other good foods include:

- Flaxseeds can help balance shifting hormones during the perimenopause, and they also contain omega 3 fatty acids, which fight depression, reduce inflammation and hot flushes and the risk of heart disease.

- Fruit and vegetables that are rich in phytoestrogens, such as soya, legumes, celery, fennel and parsley, will help to regulate oestrogen levels. Phytoestrogens have also been show to decrease in cholesterol levels, improve menopausal symptoms, reduce the risk of osteoporosis and decrease the risk of breast cancer.

- Foods rich in vitamins C and E are also important to support the body through the perimenopause.

- Two to three portions of calcium-rich foods every day (see page 27). Calcium and vitamin D are essential for bone health and to reduce the risk of osteoporosis, because bone density decreases during the menopause.

- Cruciferous veg such as broccoli, cauliflower, cabbage, kale and rocket can help your liver with detoxifying oestrogen.

Maintaining a healthy body weight also has a beneficial effect on menopausal symptoms, and in addition to sticking to a healthy diet, it is also important to take regular moderate exercise, especially weight-bearing activity (see page 53), to maintain muscle and bone strength, on two or more days each week.

FACT

Osteoporosis is a bone disease that affects over three million people in the UK. Women are at more risk of osteoporosis as they enter the menopause, but one in five men break a bone after the age of 50 because of low bone strength.

Diabetes

There are two distinct types of diabetes, and although they develop for different reasons, a healthy diet is important for people with both types and can even prevent Type 2 diabetes.

- Type 1 diabetes is the less-common form of diabetes that develops before the age of 30, when the pancreas stops producing insulin. It has to be managed with daily injections of insulin for the rest of the person's life.

- Type 2 diabetes is more common and is on the increase as obesity rates rise, Diabetes UK estimate that if we don't start to change our diets, by 2030 there will be five million people in the UK who have this form of diabetes. The good news is that is not dependent on insulin and often develops in later life. Current research suggests it can be controlled, and even avoided or reversed through healthy eating and exercise.

The recommended dietary guidelines for diabetics are essentially the same as for anyone who wants to live a healthy lifestyle – eating a nutritious diet and taking regular exercise. This enables you to manage your weight, blood glucose, blood pressure and blood cholesterol levels. In essence, diabetics are advised to eat less sugar and fat, include more fibre-rich and wholegrain foods in their diet – such as brown rice, wholegrain bread and pasta – eat plenty of fruit and vegetables and to eat moderate amounts of meat, fish, milk and dairy produce.

Tips for eating with diabetes

- **Be careful with your carbs:** Choose healthier sources that don't make your blood-sugar levels soar – reduce intake of white bread, white rice, sugary snacks and processed foods. This is particularly important for those with Type 1 diabetes.

- **Seek out sugar:** Cutting out sugar from the obvious places such as cakes, biscuits and sweets is one thing, but keep an eye out for hidden sugar, which can be included in processed foods, cereals, breads, fruit (as fructose), pizza, pasta sauces and even rice and potatoes.

- **Trim the fat:** Cut away fat from meat and use leaner cuts; use spray oil in cooking to reduce the amount you are using, or bake, steam or grill goods instead. Use healthier fats, such as olive, rapeseed or mustard-seed oil. Choose lower-fat yoghurt, cheese, cream or milk.

- **Swap out meat:** Reduce the amount of red and processed meat in your diet and replace these with poultry, eggs, fish, pulses and nuts. Oily fish such as salmon, mackerel, sardines and pilchards are particularly beneficial, because they are rich in omega 3 oils.

- **Eat the rainbow:** Try to eat more fruit and veg with meals or as snacks.

- **Drink alcohol sensibly:** Alcohol is high in calories and sugar, which will affect blood-sugar levels.

What is the glycaemic index?

You might have heard doctors and nutritionists talk about eating foods with a low glycaemic index (GI), but what does this mean? Essentially, this ranks carbohydrates as to how much sugar they produce during digestion. All breads and cereals have a high GI, whereas green veg and eggs have a low GI. Diabetics should opt for low-GI foods.

Love your heart

Heart disease is the leading cause of death worldwide, but it is also an illness that can be prevented by changing your lifestyle to include regular exercise, avoiding smoking and by eating a heart-healthy diet.

Blood pressure, cholesterol levels and other heart-disease risk factors are all affected by what you eat. Diets high in fibre, healthy fats and antioxidants have been shown to help support heart health, whereas those that include large amounts of added sugar and processed meats are associated with an increased risk of heart disease. A high-fat diet can lead to a hardening of the arteries (atherosclerosis), which will increase your risk of a heart attack. Continuing to eat high-fat foods causes fatty plaques to build up in your arteries. This is because fatty foods contain an unhealthy type of cholesterol.

There are two main types of cholesterol:

- Low-density lipoprotein (LDL) is often known as bad cholesterol because it is mostly made up of fat plus a small amount of protein, and it can block your arteries.

- High-density lipoprotein (HDL) is often known as good cholesterol because it is mostly made up of protein plus a small amount of fat, and it can reduce deposits in your arteries.

Avoid foods containing high levels of saturated fat, as they increase the amount of LDL cholesterol in your blood, and try to follow a Mediterranean-style diet, which means eating fresh food and avoiding processed foods. Try to incorporate plenty of fruit and vegetables, more oily fish, such as herring, sardines and salmon, and less meat, and reduce the amount of dairy you eat, replacing butter and cheese with products based on vegetable and plant oil, such as olive oil. Include plenty of starchy foods, too, such as bread, rice, potatoes and pasta, but choose wholegrain varieties wherever possible.

Try to reduce the amount of salt in your diet – either additional or hidden. Salt can increase the risk of developing high blood pressure.

Eating for allergies

It is estimated that up to 50 per cent of children in Britain have some form of food allergy or intolerance. While not all of these are permanent, because many either lessen or disappear as children grow up, they do require certain considerations when cooking. If you think you have an allergy or intolerance, make sure you get a medical opinion to determine the severity, and for the best advice as to how it should be managed.

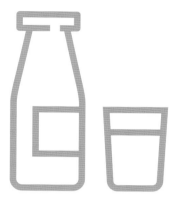

Gluten-free

Gluten is the protein component found in wheat, rye and barley and can either cause a reaction in the body (allergy or intolerance) or trigger the body's immune system to attack itself, which is a more serious and uncomfortable condition known as coeliac disease.

Found in: Any wheat-based products – bread, pasta, breakfast cereals, flour, pastry, cakes and biscuits. It can also be found in processed foods, such as soups, sauces, ready meals and sausages, and some oats can become cross contaminated during production. If you are a coeliac, make sure you buy specifically labelled gluten-free oats. Grains and cereals such as quinoa, teff, amaranth, polenta, buckwheat, corn, millet and tapioca are naturally gluten-free, as are buckwheat or rice pasta or rice noodles.

Dairy

People suffering from a dairy allergy might find they are allergic or intolerant to different ingredients. An allergy to cow's milk is an immune response to proteins such as albumin, casein or whey; while lactose intolerance is a reaction to a sugar found in cow's milk. If you exclude dairy from your diet, make sure you provide your body with calcium and iodine from other sources, such as green leafy vegetables, nuts, pulses, wholegrains, fish and fortified plant-based milks.

Found in: Milk, butter and vegetable spreads, buttermilk, yoghurt, fromage frais, cream, cheese, ice cream, custard, batter, sauces, chocolate. Try eating goat's, sheep's and buffalo milk and cheese, yoghurt and butter made from these instead. Also try plant-based milks make from soya, coconut, rice and oats.

Nuts

People who have nut allergies often have a reaction to a specific nut, but may be able to tolerate others, so it is important to get a professional diagnosis for this allergy so that you know exactly what to avoid. Nut allergies can often cause an anaphylactic reaction, which can be fatal in some cases, so it is an allergy that needs to be very carefully monitored.

Found in: Peanuts and peanut oil are used in a huge number of processed foods, such as sweets, biscuits, cakes, breakfast cereals and breads as well as takeaways and fast food. Most products should clearly state nuts as an allergen, but always read the labels of foods for nuts or traces of them to be sure.

Allergen labelling

All packaged food in the UK is covered by a law on allergen labelling, so you should be able to find out whether or not a product is safe for someone suffering an allergy or intolerance by reading the ingredients list. Wheat, cream or nuts must be listed in the ingredients and should be highlighted to stand out from other ingredients. If the food product has been made in a factory where those allergens are used in other products, the packaging may also list the allergens separately, possibly with a disclaimer stating: May contain.... But don't just take the label's word for it, always read the ingredients list carefully to see if there are any hidden allergens, and if in doubt - ask.

INGREDIENTS
Water, Carrots, Onions, Red Lentils (45%), Potatoes, Leeks, Peas, Cornflower, **Wheat** flour, Cream (**milk**), Yeast Extract, Concentrated Tomato Paste, Garlic, Sugar, **Celery** seed, Sunflower Oil, Herb and Spice, White Pepper, Parsley
ALLERGY ADVICE
For allergens, see ingredients in **bold**

Vegan or vegetarian?

Following a plant-based diet is becoming ever more popular, and some people choose to exclude meat, poultry and sometimes fish either for health reasons or out of concern for the environment.

A vegetarian diet eliminates meat, poultry and fish but usually includes eggs and dairy, however, a vegan diet is more restrictive and rules out all foods that derive from animals in any form, including dairy products, eggs, gelatine and often honey.

Removing animal products from your diet does require a little thought and research, to make sure that you are not excluding vital nutrients that your body needs. These include:

- **Protein:** All the essential amino acids are found together in meat (see page 23), so if you are following a plant-based diet you need to make sure that you are combining key sources to get all the necessary protein – eat a combination of wholegrains and legumes such as lentils, peas, soya, beans and quinoa.

- **Vitamins:** Deficiencies of vitamins B12 and D are very common, but vitamin D can be obtained from sunlight or supplements, and it is often added to breakfast cereals. Vitamin B12 can be found in breakfast cereals, soya milks and yeast extract.

- **Iron:** This can be found in many green leafy vegetables, such as cabbage and broccoli, or try fortified breakfast cereals, muesli, wholemeal bread, beans and pulses, tofu, nuts and pumpkin and sunflower seeds.

- **Calcium:** Can be found in leafy green vegetables (but not spinach), bread and foods containing brown flour, nuts, sesame seeds, tofu, pulses or fortified plant-based milks.

WELLBEING

Changing your diet is just one part of creating a happier and healthier you. Every element of your life contributes to your wellbeing – what you eat, how much exercise you take, how much sleep you get and how you manage stress.

It is important to maintain both physical and mental fitness for optimum wellbeing; these are often overlooked in the rush and demands of modern lifestyles. Once again, a healthy diet plays its part here; poor nutritional habits will make it harder for your body to reach peak performance, as it isn't being supported nutritionally to do what it needs to do.

Exercise has innumerable physical as well as psychological benefits, including improved fitness and heart health, greater body strength, better weight management, improved sleep and reduced stress, so it's a gateway to better overall health. If you have a fairly sedentary lifestyle, it is important to change the way you view physical activity so that you don't see it as something you 'have to do', 'should do' or 'ought to do' for your health, but rather as something that you do because you enjoy it and can really see its positive benefits.

The good news is, you don't have to commit to a daily gym workout or running 5k a day to keep your body healthy – unless you want to! The government's recommended guidelines for exercise is to aim to be physically active every day, to achieve a total target of at least 150 minutes of moderate intensity activity a week or 75 minutes of vigorous intensity activity a week, including strengthening activities that work all the major muscles (legs, hips, back, abdomen, chest, shoulders and arms) on at least two days a week. There is no set requirement for how much you do each day – you could do several short sessions of very vigorous intensity activity or a mix of moderate, vigorous and very vigorous intensity activity.

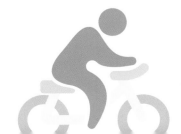

What sort of exercise should I do?

Your body is designed to be active and will perform at its optimum level if you can keep it moving. The important thing to do when exercising is to make sure that the type and intensity of the activity you choose to do is appropriate for your level of fitness, and that whatever you take part in is something you enjoy, because that will make it easier to stick to your goals.

Decide, too, whether you'd prefer to be active at home or whether you fancy a change of scenery and would prefer to get out of the house and exercise in a different environment, indoors or outdoors. Start gently, perhaps with a brisk walk every day for 10 minutes, then build up to walking or jogging for longer, or joining an exercise class. If possible, try to rotate your types of exercise so that you are supporting all elements of your physical health and to keep exercising varied and different.

There are three main types of exercise:

Cardiovascular: This is aerobic exercise that encourages the heart to work harder, beating faster to pump more blood around the body. This helps to keep heart and lungs strong, and reduces your risk of heart attacks and stroke. It also burns calories and fat, which helps you to maintain a healthy weight. It is the best kind of exercise for improving mental health, as it stimulates the release of the happy hormone, serotonin. Good forms of cardiovascular exercise include brisk walking, jogging, cycling, swimming and skipping.

Strength: Also known as resistance or weight training, this form of exercise builds and maintains muscle strength. Strength training will increase your ratio of muscle to fat, so that you burn calories and tone your physique rather than become overly muscular. It is also important for reducing natural muscle loss that you experience as you age. Good forms of strength training include lifting and exercising with free weights and resistance bands, press-ups and pull-ups, squats and lunges, and crunches or sit-ups.

Flexibility: This can be a more gentle form of exercise that helps to improve balance and coordination, and can help to relieve stress and aid relaxation. Pilates and yoga are the most popular forms, which will help to improve posture and maintain movement and flexibility, especially as you get older.

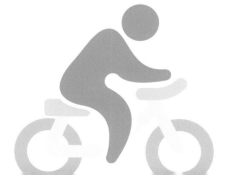

Make time for exercise

Decide how much time you have available for exercise. Don't make excuses as to why you can't do it, and plan your exercise into your week to make it easier to stick to. You may need to rejig commitments to make room for extra activities, or choose something that fits into your busy schedule or can be done around your lunch hour or work hours. If you need more motivation, book into a class or a regular series of classes, or exercise with friends or family to make it more of a sociable event.

Make exercise part of your daily life

If you're put off by sporty exercises, or don't feel inspired at the thought of limiting yourself to just one activity, remember there are lots of everyday things you can do that will get you up and active.

- **AT HOME:** The Covid-19 lockdown taught us all that you can exercise at home, and people got very creative! There is a huge range of online exercise classes out there that you can join in from the comfort of your sitting room. Lots of domestic jobs will raise your heart rate and get you off the sofa, even simple ones like pushing the lawnmower with extra vigour or putting some elbow grease into the housework.

- **AT WORK:** If you have a job that keeps you at your desk for most of the day, make sure you take regular breaks and get moving. If you work from home, get up from your chair and move around as you take phone calls. In the office, take the stairs instead of the lift, use your lunch hour to take a brisk walk, do an exercise class or go for a swim, walk or cycle to or from work, or just get off the bus or train one stop early and walk the rest of the way. The fresh air will do you good, too.

- **OUT AND ABOUT:** Getting into the fresh air and sunshine for 15 minutes a day will boost your vitamin D levels and research suggests that doing physical activity in an outdoor, 'green' environment has positive effects on mental health and mood. If you need motivation, offer to take a friend's dog out for a walk.

FACT

Just 30 minutes of brisk walking five days a week can help with weight loss, muscle strength and improve your heart and lung fitness.

Getting started

If you're new to exercising, it's not uncommon to put up some barriers to getting started. Try not to use the cost of classes or gym membership, injury, illness, lack of energy, fear of failure, or even the weather to prevent you getting going. If you are are overweight or uncomfortable with the way you look, body image can also prevent you getting out there and getting active. If this is a concern, try exercising with friends or people you trust, or wear baggier clothes until you feel more confident.

Social support is a great motivator; sharing your experiences, goals and achievements with someone else will help you to keep focus and enthusiasm. Avoid exercise studios that have mirrors in them or glass walls, so you don't feel like you're on show.

The important thing is to get started – the more you exercise the more confident you will become. Don't forget, you won't see improvement from exercise overnight, so the key is to make it a regular part of your new routine for life. Set yourself some short-term targets to help you to get to your long-term goals. Keep a record of all your activity and review it regularly so you can see your progress. There are many apps that you can download for free to help you, or try using a pedometer to measure the amount of steps you've walked or your speed and distance travelled.

Remember, making the commitment to regular physical activity is an achievement in itself, and every activity session can improve your mood.

You can't outrun bad habits

Following an exercise plan does not give you free licence to reach for the doughnuts. The saying 'You can't outrun bad habits' is true – you may burn calories when you exercise, but you can't rid your body of unhealthy foods in the process, and you can't burn all the calories you've consumed. Even an intense workout when you burn 500 calories won't counteract the 1000 calories from that pizza you ate last night!

Mental health

Managing your mental wellbeing is vital for a healthy life. It's not about being happy all the time, as it's a part of normal life to experience negative or painful emotions, such as grief, loss, or failure. It is important to feel good about ourselves, though, as people with low self-esteem often have poor relationships with food, which can lead to binge-eating and eating disorders. We all need to be able to deal with the ups and downs of life, to cope with challenges and embrace new opportunities, to feel connected to others and feel valued, and to maintain healthy relationships with others. If you are struggling with your mental health and it is impacting the way you live your life, talk to your doctor and seek help.

FACT

Around one in five adults experienced some form of depression in early 2021, more than double the number before the Covid-19 pandemic. Younger adults and women were more likely to experience some form of depression in this period, with four in ten reporting symptoms.

Exercise for mental health

Physical activity has been shown to prevent the development of mental health problems and to improve the quality of life of people who are suffering from mental health problems. Everybody experiences stress and anxiety at some point in their lives, and there can even be situations that crop up in everyday life that cause us to feel overwhelmed, but it's how we cope with these that determines how they affect our mental health and wellbeing.

Stress and anxiety is the body's reaction to feeling threatened or under pressure. When we feel these emotions it triggers a rush of stress hormones in our body – otherwise known as the 'fight or flight' response. These hormones, known as adrenaline and noradrenaline, raise the blood pressure, increase the heart rate and the rate at which we perspire, preparing our body to urgently respond to the threat. They can also reduce blood flow to our skin and our stomach, while cortisol, another stress hormone, releases fat and sugar into the system to boost our energy. The most common physical signs of stress include sleeping problems, sweating and loss of appetite. While low-level stress can sometimes be motivational, severe and unrelenting stress can be detrimental to physical and mental health.

Physical activity has been shown to have a positive impact on our mood. Even a brisk 10-minute walk boosts our energy and mood. Regular physical activity can also increase self-esteem and reduce stress and anxiety, and if done in a group setting it can create a sense of community and camaraderie, too, which can be vital for those living on their own, or people who struggle to get out much to socialise.

As well as providing another focus for our overwhelmed brains and distracting us from our worries, getting active also improves the body's ability to use oxygen and blood flow, which has a beneficial impact on the brain.

Feeling depressed can have a huge impact on your physical health as well as your mental health. The condition can leave you feeling very low in energy and less inclined to get active, or you might feel that you can't face going out, which can restrict your options for activities. However, it is important to exercise, to trigger the brain's production of those all-important endorphins, which are the 'feel-good' neurotransmitters that give you a sense of wellbeing and euphoria and boost the mood.

Getting out and moving can also help you to break the cycle of negative thoughts that can feed depression. Exercise can boost our self-esteem, which can improve our ability to cope with the stresses of life. It also has the added benefit of helping you sleep better at night, so there really is nothing to lose.

Stress and digestion

The effects of stress on our eating habits and digestion can lead to fluctuations in appetite and digestive problems such as irritable bowel syndrome. This is because the fight or flight response in the central nervous system shuts down digestion, restricting blood flow, slowing the contractions of the digestive muscles and decreasing the secretions needed for the digestive process. The body does this so it can prioritise more important functions, such as increasing heart and breathing rates to prepare the body to attack or escape a threat.

After a stressful period, the body goes into recovery mode, where the appetite increases and food cravings can take hold. At the same time, metabolic rates drop to conserve energy, and the body is prone to storing fat – particularly around the abdomen. Feeling stressed can lead to an increase in levels of cortisol, a hormone that contributes to weight gain. Chronic stress can lead to weight loss by suppressing the appetite, so our bodies rely on existing energy stores to operate effectively.

Dementia and cognitive decline

Dementia is a progressive disease that results in memory loss and a decline in cognitive functions, such as attention and concentration, that occurs in older people. For people who have already developed dementia, studies have shown that physical activity can help to delay further decline in function and lowers the risk of depression and dementia by 20–30%.

Vitamin D and mental health

Vitamin D is as vital for mental health as it is for physical health, and it is thought that it plays an important role in regulating mood. A deficiency of vitamin D has been linked to depression and Seasonal Affective Disorder (SAD), because the body acquires this vitamin through sunlight. In fact, people suffereing from a vitamin D deficiency experience similar symptoms to those suffering from depression:

- Mood changes accompanied by overwhelming feelings of hopelessness and sadness
- Feeling exhausted
- Forgetfulness
- Loss of interest in previously enjoyable activities
- Isolation and withdrawal
- Anxiety
- Loss of appetite
- Excessive weight loss or gain
- Trouble sleeping

You cannot overdose on vitamin D through exposure to sunlight, so try to get outside at least once a day. Always remember to cover up or protect your skin if you're out in the sun for long periods, in order to reduce the risk of skin damage and skin cancer.

Embracing mindfulness

It's so easy to rush through our daily lives and get so caught up in our everyday tasks that we fail to notice the impact this is having on our emotions and behaviour.

Becoming more aware of the present moment can help us to enjoy the world around us more, to understand ourselves better, and positively change the way we see ourselves and our lives. It allows us to experience afresh things that we have been taking for granted.

Paying more attention to the present moment – reconnecting with our bodies, our own thoughts and feelings and the world around us – can improve our mental wellbeing by helping us to reframe our thoughts and identify unhelpful patterns of thinking. This can in turn help us let go of these negative thoughts and deal better with difficult situations.

How to be more mindful

Remind yourself every day to take a moment to notice your thoughts, your feelings and the sensations in your body.

- Pick a regular time of day to practise mindfulness, if necessary, set an alarm or a reminder on your phone to take time out.

- Take a walk and leave your phone at home – raise your eyes from the ground and look up to experience a new view of your local area.

- Be aware of your thoughts, when negative thoughts or worries enter your mind, acknowledge them and dismiss them.

- Try meditation. Stop what you are doing – set a timer if need be – close your eyes and relax your shoulders and switch off from everything around you. Deepen your breathing and regulate it so that it is even, in and out. Do this for 3–5 minutes and try to focus simply on the act of breathing. Empty your mind.

The importance of sleep

Sleep is vital for physical and mental wellbeing – a good night's sleep can see you jumping out of bed refreshed and energised, while a bad night's sleep can be debilitating the next day and have you reaching for sugar-filled foods for an instant energy boost.

The odd broken night of sleep is bearable, but if it becomes a regular occurrence it can have serious consequences for your health and you should see a doctor. The body and brain need time to recover and restore function to nearly every tissue in the body. Sleep deprivation increases the risk of health conditions like diabetes, heart disease and stroke. Prolonged sleep deprivation can also affect concentration and other cognitive functions, making previously manageable tasks much more difficult. It has also been seen to have a significant link to depression and poor mental health.

How we sleep and how much sleep we need is different for all of us and changes as we get older, but the NHS guidance suggests that most adults need on average at least seven to nine hours of sleep a night. Not getting enough sleep also has a significant impact on physical health, because you won't have the energy to exercise during the day. However, getting regular exercise can improve sleep quality – and any amount of movement can help.

There is an important link between sleep and food, too; the more tired you are, the more you tend to overeat and choose unhealthy foods, because exhaustion produces hunger hormones. As a result of poor diet and lack of exercise, chronic sleep loss can often lead to obesity.

What we eat also impacts sleep quality and duration. Caffeine and alcohol are both stimulants and if drunk in the evening can make it more difficult to fall asleep, as can eating too close to bedtime.

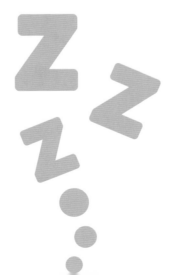

Tips for better sleep

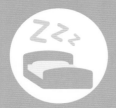

- Keep a regular bedtime – go to bed when you feel tired in the evening and don't force yourself to stay awake. Try to avoid napping during the day.

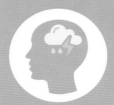

- Create a restful environment – make sure the room is dark, quiet, clutter-free and at a cool temperature. Keep mobile phones out of the bedroom, too, as LED screens emit a blue light that can inhibit the production of the sleep-inducing hormone melatonin.

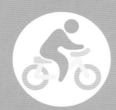

- Get active during the day, but avoid exercising just before bedtime, as this will increase stress hormones, which can make sleep difficult.

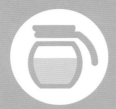

- Avoid drinking caffeine or alcohol in the evening as these can make it harder to fall asleep and stay asleep.

- If you are lying in bed awake, rather than worry about not sleeping, get up and move around, then go back to bed when you feel sleepy.

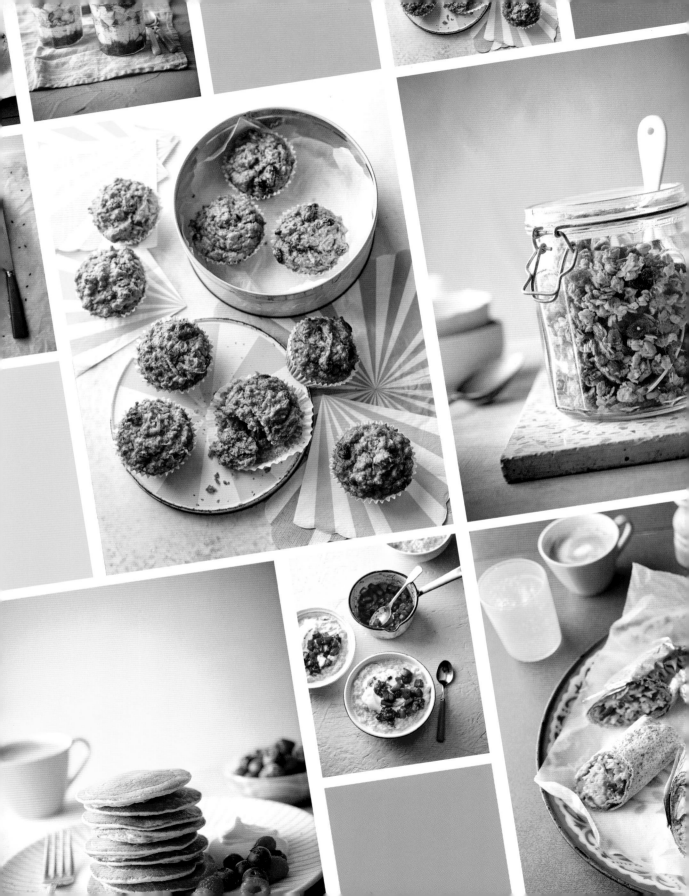

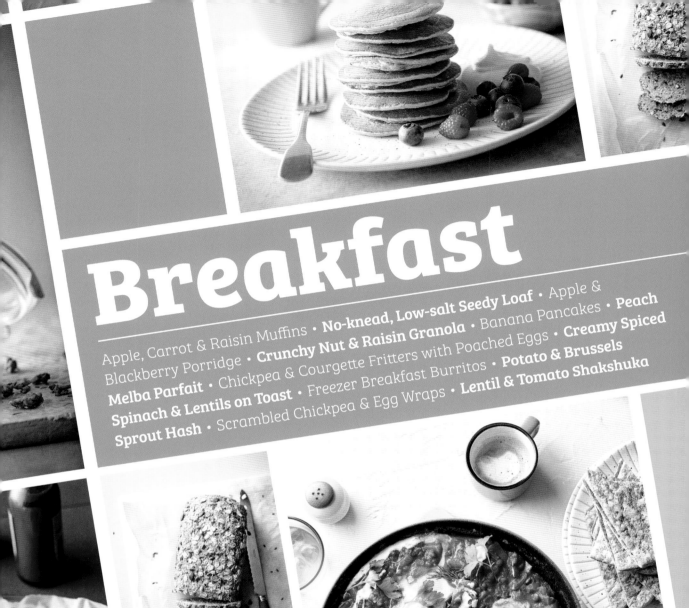

Breakfast

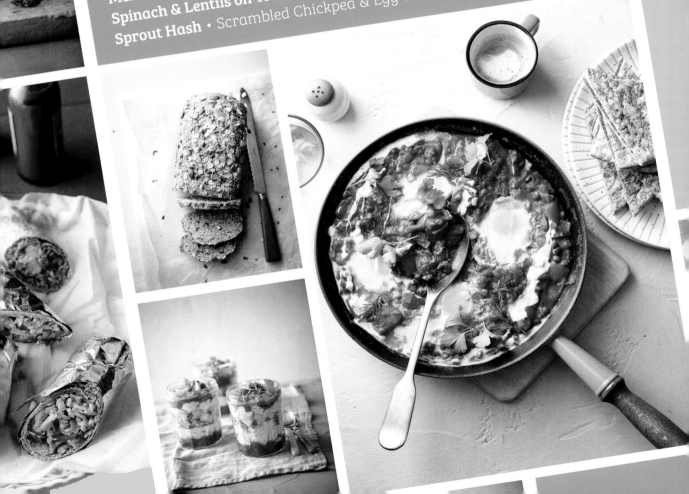

Apple, Carrot & Raisin Muffins

These fruity spiced muffins use apples, carrots, olive oil and almonds to make a naturally sweet, fibre-packed and low-sugar breakfast or snack that will keep you going all morning.

MAKES 10 • 10 MINS • 27 MINS •

3 eating apples (420g), coarsely grated

1 medium carrot (120g), coarsely grated

120ml extra virgin olive oil

120ml milk

50g granulated sugar

2 large eggs, beaten

1½ tsp ground cinnamon

120g plain wholemeal flour

80g porridge oats

50g ground almonds

1½ tsp baking powder

½ tsp bicarbonate of soda

75g raisins

1. Preheat the oven to 200°C/180°C fan/400°F/gas mark 6 and line 10 cups of a standard muffin tin with paper liners.

2. Place the grated apples and carrot onto a clean tea towel, gather the edges at the top and twist them together to make a bundle. Squeeze over the sink to remove as much of the liquid as possible then unwrap and tip into a large bowl.

3. Mix in the oil, milk, sugar, eggs and cinnamon until combined. Add the flour, oats, ground almonds, baking powder and bicarbonate of soda, then stir until no floury patches remain. Finally, fold in the raisins. The batter should be thick.

4. Divide the batter between the paper liners, filling them to the top. Bake for 22–27 minutes or until a toothpick inserted into the centre of a muffin comes out clean.

5. Remove from the tin and allow to cool on a wire rack completely before storing in an airtight container for up to 4 days. The muffins can also be frozen in a sealed sandwich bag for up to 3 months.

TIPS

If you don't like raisins, leave them out or replace them with an equal weight of your favourite dried fruit.

If using larger dried fruits, such as apricots or dates, roughly chop them before adding to the batter.

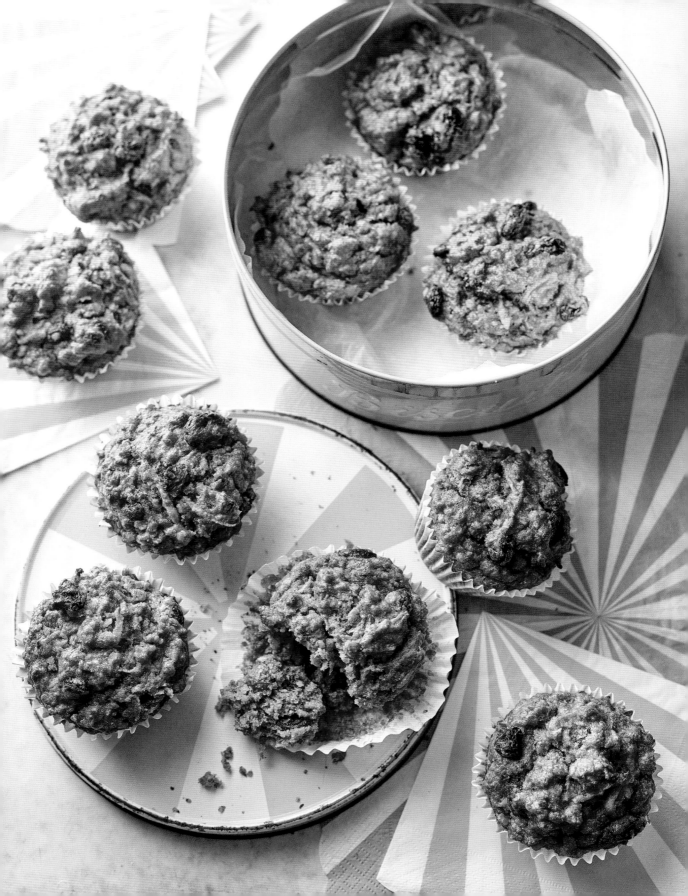

No-knead, Low-salt Seedy Loaf

This loaf needs rising time, so prepare it in advance, but as it freezes well, you can slice it and store it ready for use. There's no salt, but the seeds and wholemeal flour add a nutty flavour.

MAKES A 900G LOAF • 10 MINS, PLUS PROVING • 50 MINS •

280g wholemeal bread flour

80g porridge oats, plus a sprinkling for the top

½ tsp fast-action yeast

280g warm water

120g natural yoghurt

30g sunflower seeds

30g pumpkin seeds

20g sesame seeds

2 tbsp linseeds

1. Combine the flour, oats and yeast in a large bowl and mix briefly to combine. Pour in the water and yoghurt and stir with a wooden spoon to make a sticky dough. Beat with a spoon for 1 minute. Cover the bowl with a piece of cling film and leave in a warm place for 5 hours.

2. Uncover the bowl and mix in all the seeds. Scrape into a greased, lined 900g loaf tin, evenly sprinkle the top with some oats and leave to rise somewhere warm for 45 minutes until puffy.

3. Once the loaf has risen, preheat the oven to 200°C/180°C fan/400°F/gas mark 6. Bake for 40–50 minutes until evenly golden on top. Allow to cool in the tin for 10 minutes before tipping out onto a wire rack to cool completely.

TIPS

This loaf freezes well. Once cold, slice and wrap in baking parchment before packing into a freezer bag and popping in the freezer. Slicing it first means you can defrost a slice at a time.

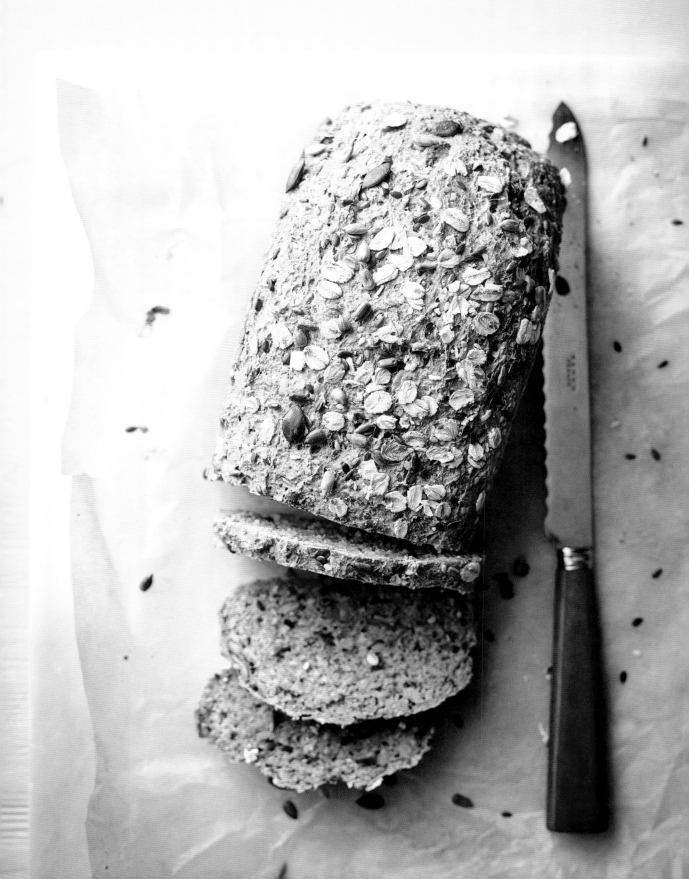

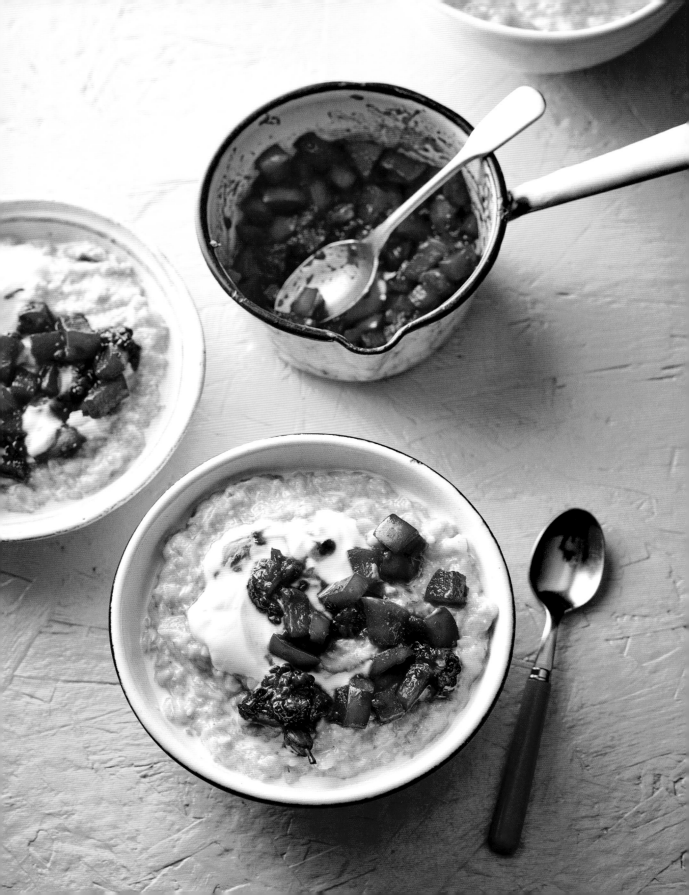

Apple & Blackberry Porridge

Oats are an excellent source of protein and fibre to make you feel fuller for longer, so they are a great breakfast choice to keep snacks at bay, topped wth a fruity, flavoursome compote.

SERVES 4 • 10 MINS • 10 MINS • V

FOR THE PORRIDGE

2 eating apples, grated

160g jumbo oats

800ml water

Pinch of salt

Splash of milk

4 tbsp natural yoghurt, to serve

FOR THE COMPOTE

2 eating apples, cored and diced

80g blackberries

2 tbsp water

2 tsp honey

2 cardamom pods or ½ tsp ground cinnamon

1. Place the grated apples, oats, water and salt into a medium pan over a high heat on the hob. Bring to a boil then cover with a lid, remove from the heat and allow to sit for 5 minutes. Once the time is up, remove the lid and stir in a splash of milk to loosen.

2. Meanwhile, make the compote, combine the diced apples, blackberries, water and honey in a medium pan. Crush the cardamom pods with the side of a knife and add to the pan, or just sprinkle in the cinnamon. Place over a medium–low heat, cover with a lid, and leave to cook until the apples are soft – around 10 minutes. Remove from the heat and crush some of the compote with the back of a fork.

3. Divide the porridge between 4 bowls then top with the compote and the yoghurt.

Crunchy Nut & Raisin Granola

Shop-bought granola can be full of sugar, but this healthy homemade version means you can use less sugar and add your favourite ingredients to make a protein-packed, gut-healthy cereal.

SERVES 8–10 • 10 MINS • 40 MINS • Ⓥ

30g extra virgin olive oil

40g runny honey

60g aquafaba or 2 egg whites

80g mashed ripe banana or unsweetened applesauce

Pinch of salt

250g jumbo oats

50g mixed seeds (linseed, sunflower, sesame, pumpkin, hemp or poppy seeds)

50g peanuts, roughly chopped (optional)

100g raisins

1. Preheat the oven to 170°C/150°C fan/325°F/gas mark 3 and line a large, rimmed baking tray with baking paper.

2. Combine the olive oil, honey, aquafaba or egg whites, mashed banana or applesauce and salt in a large bowl. Mix until smooth then fold in the oats, seeds and peanuts, if using.

3. Spread out evenly on the lined baking tray and bake for 30–40 minutes, stirring every 10 minutes or so, until slightly golden all over. The granola may feel slightly soft when warm but should crisp up as it cools. Allow to cool on the baking tray, then stir in the raisins.

4. The granola will keep for up to 2 weeks in an airtight container.

TIPS

You can make your own applesauce; simmer peeled, cored apples in a lidded pot with a splash of water until soft – about 10–15 minutes. Blitz until smooth.

If you're allergic to peanuts, remove them or replace with extra mixed seeds.

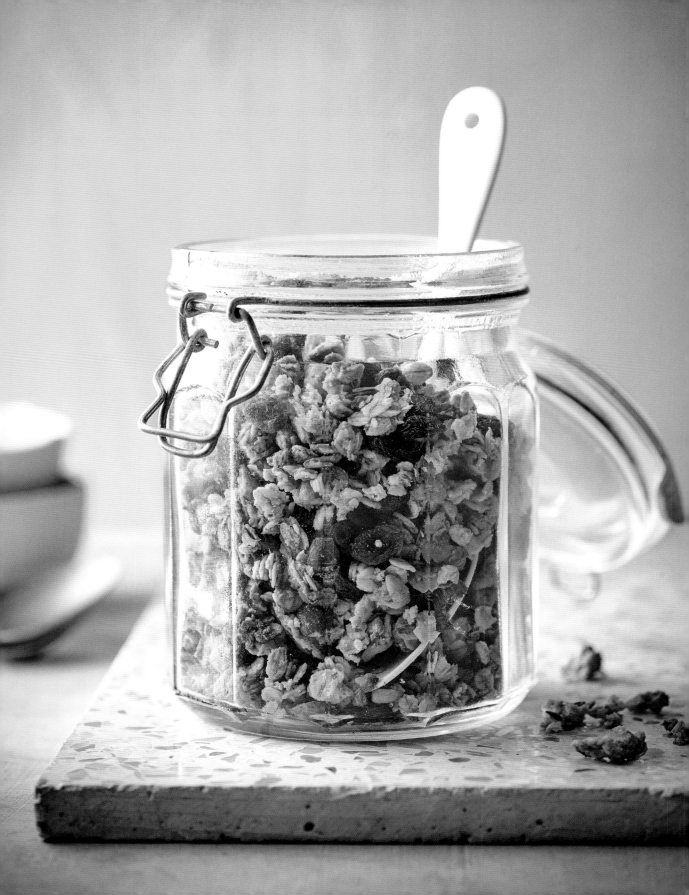

Banana Pancakes

An easy way to start the day; a protein-packed breakfast for all the family. Multiply the quantities by the number of people. Serve with fruit for extra sweetness and a nutrient boost!

SERVES 1 • 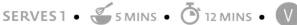 5 MINS • ⏱ 12 MINS • Ⓥ

1 large ripe banana (around 120g peeled weight)

2 large eggs

1 tbsp smooth peanut butter (or nut butter of your choice), or 1 tbsp ground almonds

TO SERVE

Natural yoghurt

Fresh berries

1. Peel the banana and put into a blender with the eggs and nut butter, blending until smooth. If you don't have a blender, use the back of a fork to mash the banana and nut butter on a plate until smooth, scrape into a bowl, then whisk in the eggs to thoroughly combine.

2. Heat a medium, non-stick frying pan over a low heat. Pour in puddles of the batter using around 2 tablespoons of batter per pancake. Leave to cook over a low heat for 1–2 minutes or until the underside has browned, then use a thin metal spatula to flip them over and cook for another 1–2 minutes or until the other side is golden. Remove to a plate and keep warm while you repeat with the remaining batter until all of it is used up – it should make 9 mini pancakes.

3. Serve the pancakes with a spoonful of natural yoghurt and some fresh berries.

TIPS

To make blueberry pancakes, dot a few fresh or frozen blueberries over the surface of the batter just after pouring it into the pan.

Add ¼ tsp baking powder to the pancake batter for a fluffier, thicker pancake.

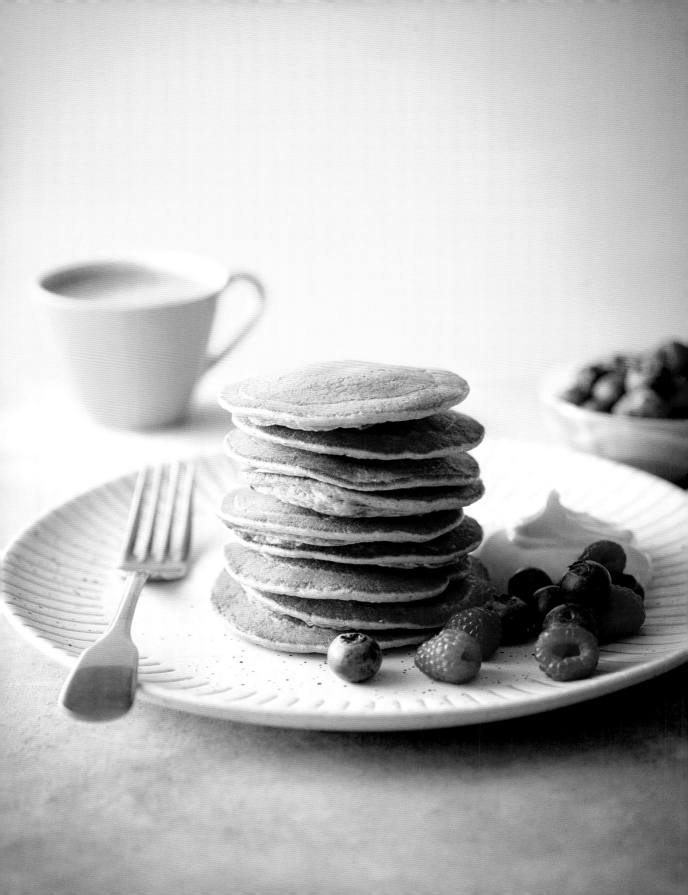

Peach Melba Parfait

A little pot of probiotic heaven for your gut! So easy to put together, this delicious combination of oats, natural yoghurt and fruit will feed both you and your beneficial gut bacteria.

SERVES 4 • 5 MINS • NONE • V

400g natural yoghurt
2 tsp vanilla extract or vanilla paste
1 tbsp chia seeds
120g fresh or frozen raspberries
1 tbsp honey
120g unsweetened muesli
4 peaches, stoned and diced

1. Stir together the yoghurt, vanilla and chia seeds in a small bowl.

2. Mash the raspberries and honey on a plate with the back of a fork.

3. In 4 wide glasses or jars, layer half the mashed raspberries followed by half of the yoghurt, half of the muesli and half of the diced peaches. Repeat the layers to use up the remaining ingredients – starting with the chia, then the raspberries, and finishing with the fruit and muesli.

4. You can chill this overnight, covered with clingfilm, or eat immediately.

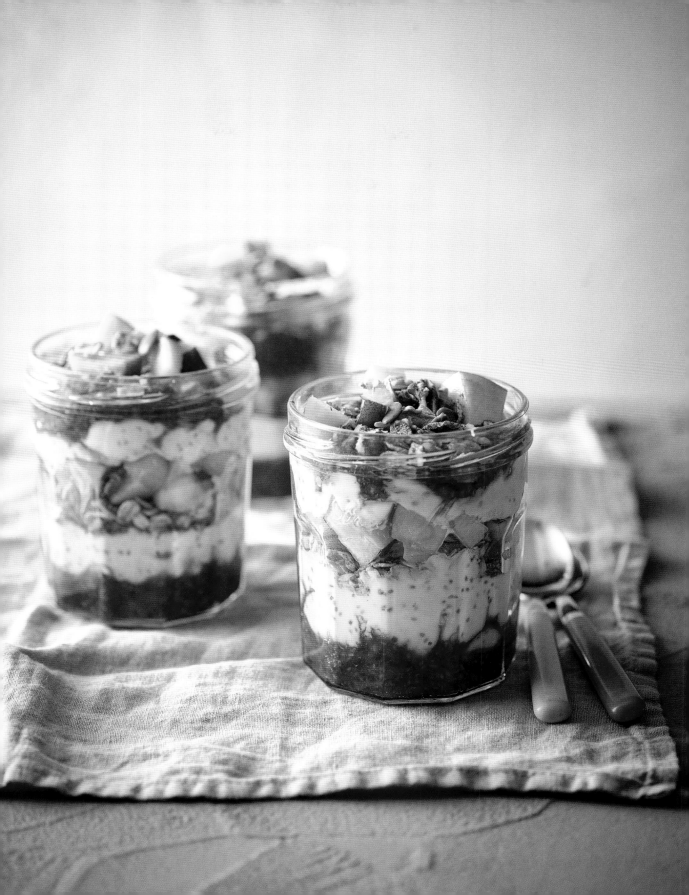

Chickpea & Courgette Fritters with Poached Eggs

A super-simple vegetable and chickpea fritter that you can have on the table quickly, or you can batch-cook and freeze. Top with eggs poached to your liking for an extra protein hit.

SERVES 4 • 10 MINS • 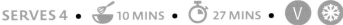 27 MINS •

2 tbsp extra virgin olive oil

1 x 400g tin chickpeas, drained and rinsed

400g courgette, coarsely grated

250g frozen sweetcorn, defrosted

250g ricotta cheese

60g dry breadcrumbs, preferably wholemeal

6 large eggs

1 green chilli, seeds removed, finely chopped

Pinch of salt

1. Preheat the oven to 180°C/160°C fan/350°F/gas mark 4, line a large baking tray with baking paper, brush with half of the oil and set aside.

2. Tip the chickpeas into a large bowl and mash slightly with a potato masher to break them down a bit.

3. Place the grated courgettes into a clean tea towel, gather the edges at the top and twist them together to make a bundle. Squeeze over the sink to remove as much of the liquid as possible then tip the grated courgette into the bowl.

4. Add the sweetcorn, ricotta, breadcrumbs, 2 of the eggs, the chilli and a pinch of salt to the bowl. Mix together until well combined. Scoop 2 heaped tablespoons of mixture onto the tray, then flatten. Repeat with the remaining mixture then drizzle with the remaining oil. Bake for 20 minutes, flipping the cakes over halfway through the cooking time. The fritters can be frozen at this point – once cold, wrap each in baking paper and pop in a freezerproof box.

5. Heat the grill and cook the cakes for 2–4 minutes, until browned on top.

6. Meanwhile, bring a deep frying pan (or wide pan) of water to the boil then turn the heat down to a very gentle simmer. Gently crack the remaining 4 eggs into the water and cook for 2½–3 minutes, until the whites are set but the yolks are runny. Remove with a slotted spoon to a plate lined with paper towel to drain.

7. Serve the corn fritters with the poached eggs on top.

Creamy Spiced Spinach & Lentils on Toast

Perk up your toast with this really easy and fast topping; a delicious way to get veg into your breakfast. Gives a boost of protein, iron and vitamins A and C thanks to the spinach and lentils.

SERVES 4 • 5 MINS • 15 MINS • 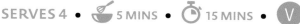 V

2 tbsp extra virgin olive oil

2 banana shallots or 2 small onions, thinly sliced

Pinch of salt

4 garlic cloves, crushed

1 x 400g tin green lentils, drained and rinsed

400g baby spinach or 300g whole-leaf frozen spinach

150g low-fat cream cheese

2 tsp curry powder

4 slices wholemeal, seeded toast, to serve

1. Heat the oil in a large, non-stick frying pan over a medium heat. Add the shallots or onions with a pinch of salt and cook until starting to turn golden – 7–10 minutes. Stir in the garlic, lentils and spinach until the spinach has all wilted down. Finally, stir in the cream cheese and curry powder until the cheese has melted and mixed through.

2. Divide between the pieces of toast and serve.

TIPS

Serve with poached eggs for a more substantial meal.

Make ahead: The lentil spinach mixture can be kept in an airtight container in the fridge for up to 3 days, then warm over a low heat in a pan.

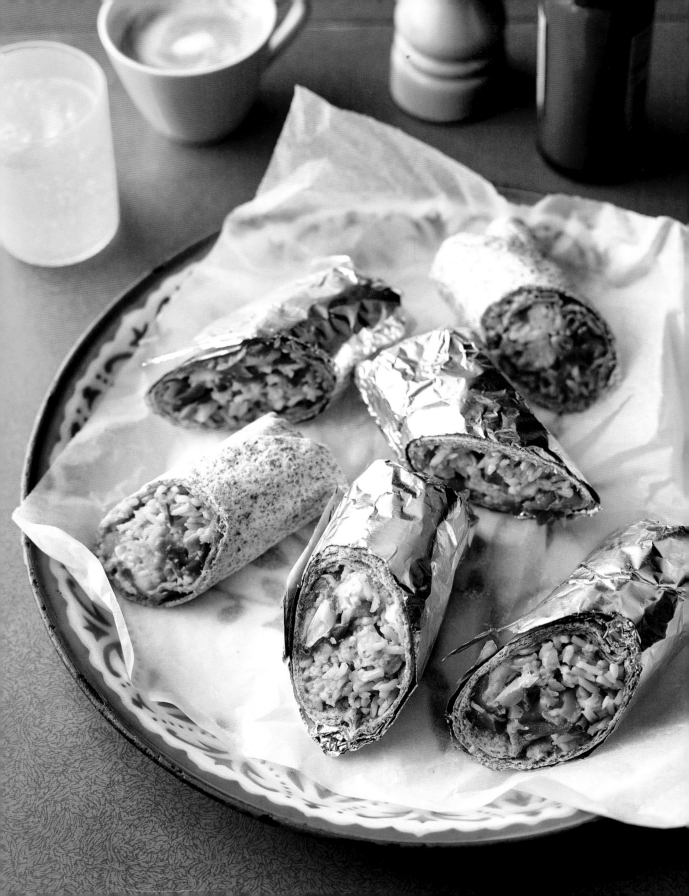

Freezer Breakfast Burritos

Brilliant for an easy breakfast – prepare ahead and either cook from frozen in the microwave or defrost overnight to oven bake. Customise these with your choice of beans, veg or spices.

SERVES 4 • 15 MINS • ⏱ 30 MINS • Ⓥ ❄

8 eggs

Pinch of salt

1 tbsp extra virgin olive oil

500g frozen sliced peppers

8 spring onions, sliced into 3cm lengths

6 wholemeal wraps

250g cooked brown rice

75g feta cheese

Hot sauce (optional)

1. Briefly whisk the eggs together with a pinch of salt in a medium bowl.

2. Heat the oil in a large, non-stick frying pan over a medium-high heat. Add the peppers and cook for about 5 minutes or until they've softened and any liquid has cooked off. Remove from the heat and pour in the beaten eggs. Stir, off the heat, letting the residual heat cook the eggs. If the eggs aren't cooked to your liking you can pop the pan back on the heat until they are. Fold in the spring onions off the heat.

3. Lay out the wraps. Divide the rice and the egg mixture between them. Crumble the feta over and top with a drizzle of hot sauce, if you like. Fold in the sides of the tortilla, then roll up into a tight log.

4. Individually wrap each burrito in a piece of tin foil. Pop them into a sandwich bag, squeeze out the air and seal the bag. Freeze for up to 3 months.

5. When you are ready to reheat the burritos, you can do this in the microwave or the oven. If you are using the microwave, remove the foil from the frozen burrito, then wrap in a damp piece of paper towel and microwave for 2–3 minutes until piping hot throughout. To cook in the oven, let the burritos defrost overnight in the fridge. Bake in an oven preheated to 200°C/180°C fan/400°F/gas mark 6 for 20–25 minutes until piping hot throughout.

Potato & Brussels Sprout Hash

Even if you think you don't like sprouts, give this a go, because when sautéed they have a sweet, nutty flavour and will give you a great vitamin K and C and fibre boost.

SERVES 4 • 15 MINS • 20 MINS •

450g floury potatoes, such as King Edward

300g Brussels sprouts, thinly sliced

2½ tbsp extra virgin olive oil

1 x 400g tin cannellini beans, drained and rinsed

1 garlic clove, crushed

4 eggs

Salt and black pepper

Peri-peri hot sauce (or hot sauce of your preference) or lemon wedges, to serve

1. Grate the potatoes on the coarse side of a box grater, toss with a pinch of salt and set aside for 5 minutes. Once the time is up, wrap in a tea towel and squeeze over the sink to remove as much liquid as possible.

2. Heat 2 tablespoons of the oil in a large, non-stick frying pan over a high heat. Once hot, sprinkle the grated potatoes into the pan, covering the entire surface. Pat down and allow to cook until golden underneath, about 5 minutes. Flip and cook until the other side is golden, about 5 minutes more – the potato hash may break when you do this but that's fine. Remove to a plate and set aside.

3. Heat the remaining oil in the same pan over a medium heat and add the sliced sprouts. Stir for 5–8 minutes until softened, then mix in the beans and garlic with a pinch of salt. Make 4 holes in the mixture and crack in the eggs, then cover the pan with a lid. Cook over a low heat until the egg whites have set but the yolks are soft.

4. Divide between 4 plates and serve with hot sauce or a squeeze of lemon juice and some black pepper.

Scrambled Chickpea & Egg Wraps

Chickpeas add a delicious crunch and punch of fibre to a breakfast favourite. Ordinarily bland scrambled eggs are made more interesting with the addition of garlic and ginger.

SERVES 4 • 10 MINS • 18 MINS • **V**

300g chestnut mushrooms, sliced

1 tsp sesame oil

1 tbsp extra virgin olive oil

350g cherry tomatoes, halved

1 x 400g tin chickpeas

2 tsp grated fresh ginger

2 garlic cloves, crushed

4 large eggs

4 spring onions, thinly sliced

Handful of fresh coriander, roughly chopped

8 small wholemeal wraps, warmed

2 tsp soy sauce, to serve

1. Add the sliced mushrooms to a large non-stick frying pan over a medium heat. Cook for about 5 minutes, until they've released their liquid and are starting to brown. Add the sesame oil, olive oil and tomatoes to the pan and cook for about 5 minutes or until the tomatoes have softened.

2. Drain the chickpeas but reserve 60ml of the liquid from the tin. Add the chickpeas and the reserved liquid to the pan and use the back of your spoon to roughly crush half of them. Stir in the ginger and garlic and cook for a minute or two until the liquid has been cooked off.

3. Turn the heat down to low, crack in the eggs and scramble them directly in the pan. Keep stirring over a low heat until they're cooked to your liking – about 2–5 minutes. Remove from the heat and fold in the spring onions and coriander. Divide between the warmed wraps, fold in the sides and roll up, then serve with the soy sauce for drizzling.

Lentil & Tomato Shakshuka

A comforting, warming breakfast or brunch, this hearty, protein-packed pan of peppers, tomatoes, lentils and eggs will set you up for a busy day and keep you fuller for longer.

SERVES 4 • 10 MINS • 20 MINS • Ⓥ

1 tbsp extra virgin olive oil

1 onion, diced

2 red peppers, deseeded and diced

Pinch of salt

1 x 400g tin green lentils, drained and rinsed

1 x 400g tin chopped tomatoes

1 tbsp balsamic vinegar

2 tsp smoked paprika

1 tsp ground cumin

4 eggs

TO SERVE

3 tbsp natural yoghurt

Handful of fresh parsley, roughly chopped

Handful of fresh dill, roughly chopped

4 wholemeal pita breads, toasted

1. Heat the oil in a large frying pan over a medium heat and sauté the onion and peppers with a pinch of salt until softened and turning golden, about 10 minutes.

2. Tip in the lentils, tomatoes, vinegar, paprika and cumin. Stir well to combine then leave to simmer for 5 minutes until slightly thickened and reduced. Taste and season with salt, as needed.

3. Make 4 wells in the tomato mixture and crack in the eggs. Turn the heat down to low, cover with a lid and leave to cook until the eggs are set to your liking.

4. Remove from the heat, garnish with the yoghurt and fresh herbs, and serve with the toasted pita.

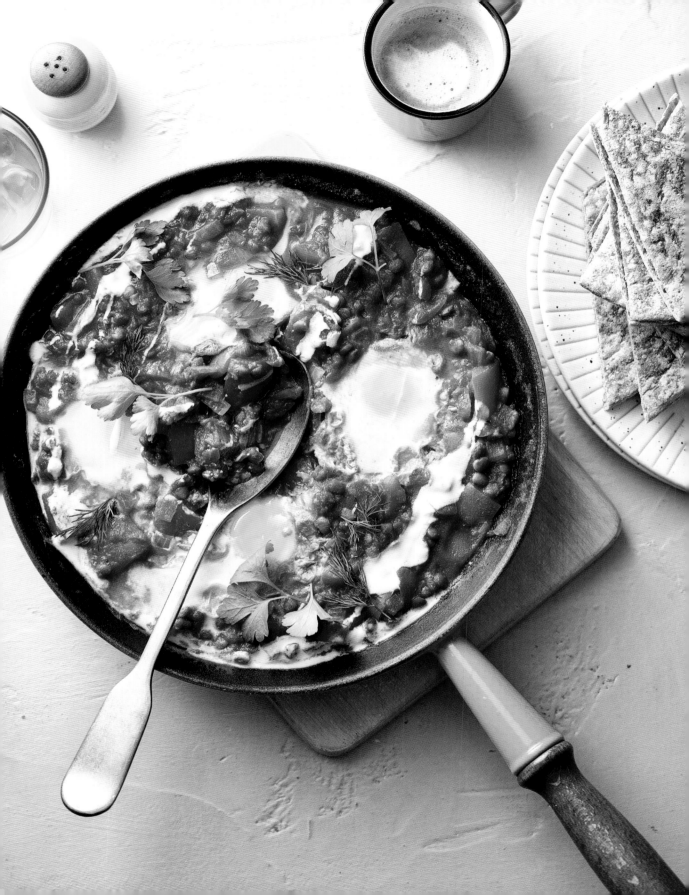

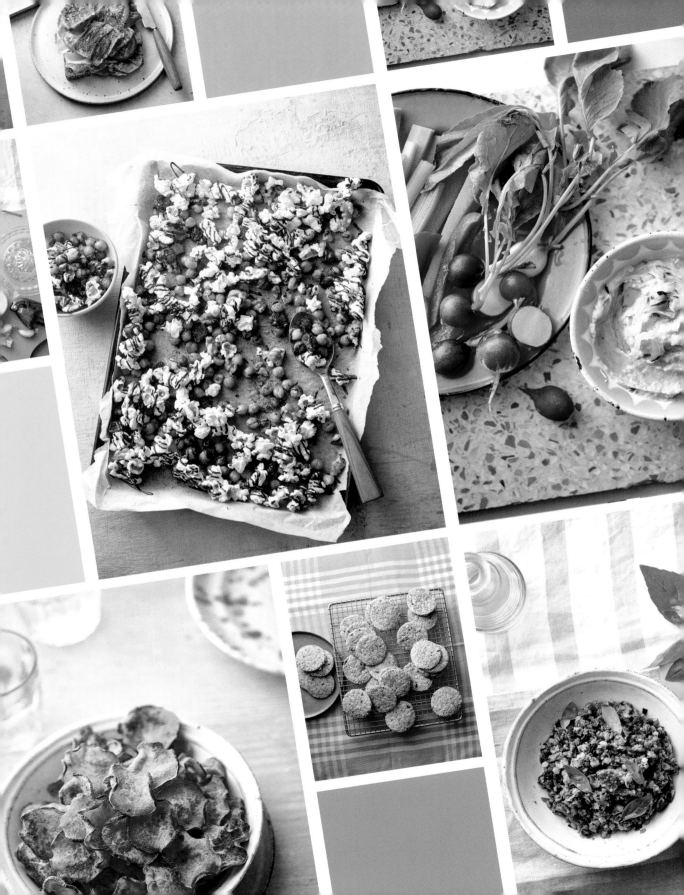

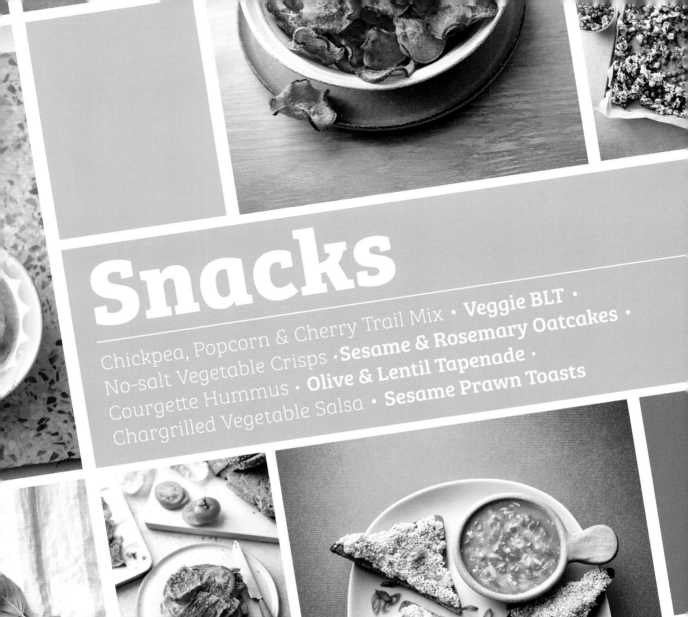

Snacks

Chickpea, Popcorn & Cherry Trail Mix • Veggie BLT • No-salt Vegetable Crisps • **Sesame & Rosemary Oatcakes** • Courgette Hummus • **Olive & Lentil Tapenade** • Chargrilled Vegetable Salsa • **Sesame Prawn Toasts**

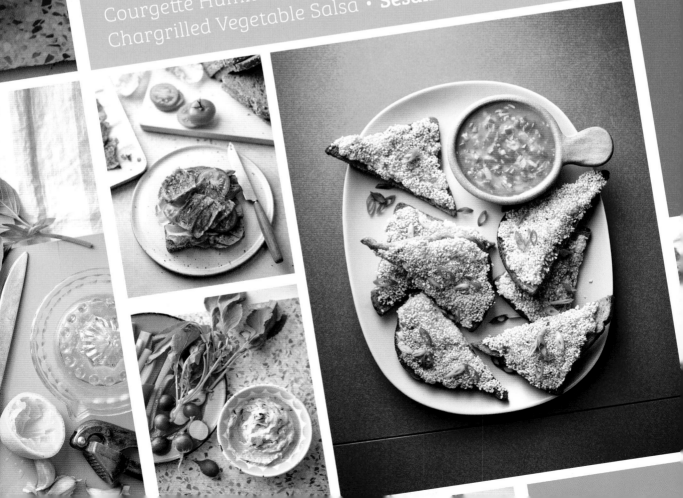

Chickpea, Popcorn & Cherry Trail Mix

If you've got a craving for chocolate, this is the perfect way to satisfy that sweet tooth – guilt free! Chickpeas and nuts add crunch, fibre and protein, drizzled with a healthy hit of dark choc.

SERVES 4 • 5 MINS • 30 MINS • V

1 x 400g tin chickpeas
1 tbsp olive oil
Pinch of salt
1 tbsp light brown sugar
½ tsp ground cinnamon
20g popped salted popcorn
30g dried cherries
40g walnut pieces
30g dark chocolate (85% cocoa solids), melted

1. Preheat the oven to 200°C/180°C fan/400°F/gas mark 6 and line a shallow rimmed baking tray with baking paper.

2. Drain but don't rinse the chickpeas. Toss with the oil and a pinch of salt on the baking tray and roast for 15 minutes. Remove from the oven and sprinkle over the sugar and cinnamon, mix and return to the oven for 10–15 minutes until light golden and crisp.

3. To the tray add the popcorn, cherries and walnuts and stir well to combine. Drizzle the chocolate all over, leave for a few minutes to allow the chocolate to set, then enjoy.

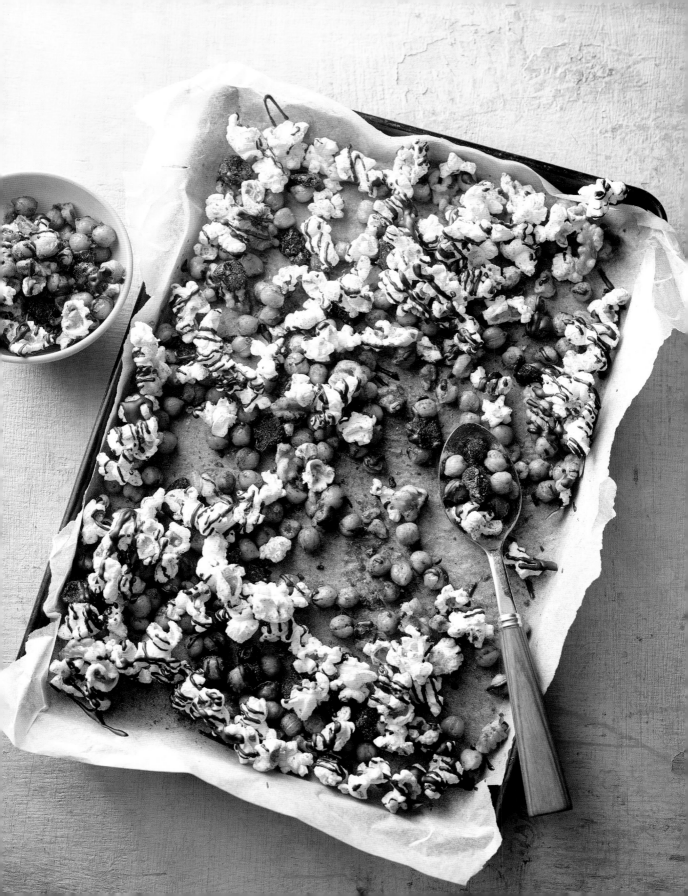

Veggie BLT

With a little advance prep, this makes a delicious, meat-free lunch in minutes.

SERVES 1 • 5 MINS • NONE •

1 tbsp mayonnaise
2 slices wholemeal or seeded bread
2 little gem lettuce leaves
1 tomato, sliced
3–4 Smoky Tofu Bacon slices
   (see recipe below)

1. Spread the mayo over one slice of bread, top with the gem lettuce, tomato and Smoky Tofu Bacon slices. Top with the second slice of bread and serve.

Smoky Tofu Bacon

A really tasty alternative to bacon for those who don't eat meat or are trying to cut back. With a smoky, meaty flavour, it's great in sandwiches, in salads or just as a snack to nibble on.

SERVES 1 • 10 MINS • 24 MINS •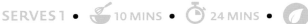

225g smoked tofu (or use plain tofu), cut into 2mm-thick slices
2 tbsp cornflour
1 tbsp extra virgin olive oil

GLAZE
1 tbsp soy sauce
½ tbsp maple syrup
1 tsp smoked paprika
½ tsp garlic granules
1 tsp tomato puree

1. Preheat the oven to 200°C/180°C fan/400°F/gas mark 6 and line a baking tray with baking paper.

2. Lay the tofu slices out over one half of a clean tea towel. Fold the other half of the towel over the slices and press down to blot the moisture from the tofu.

3. Place the cornflour in a wide, shallow dish. Dip both sides of each piece of tofu into it, tapping and shaking them to remove excess cornflour then place onto the lined baking tray. Drizzle with the olive oil and bake for 20 minutes, flipping them over halfway through.

4. Mix together all of the glaze ingredients in a small bowl. Brush the glaze over the baked tofu and return to the oven for 2 minutes. Flip the tofu slices over and brush the other side with glaze. Bake for a final 2 minutes then remove from the oven and allow to cool.

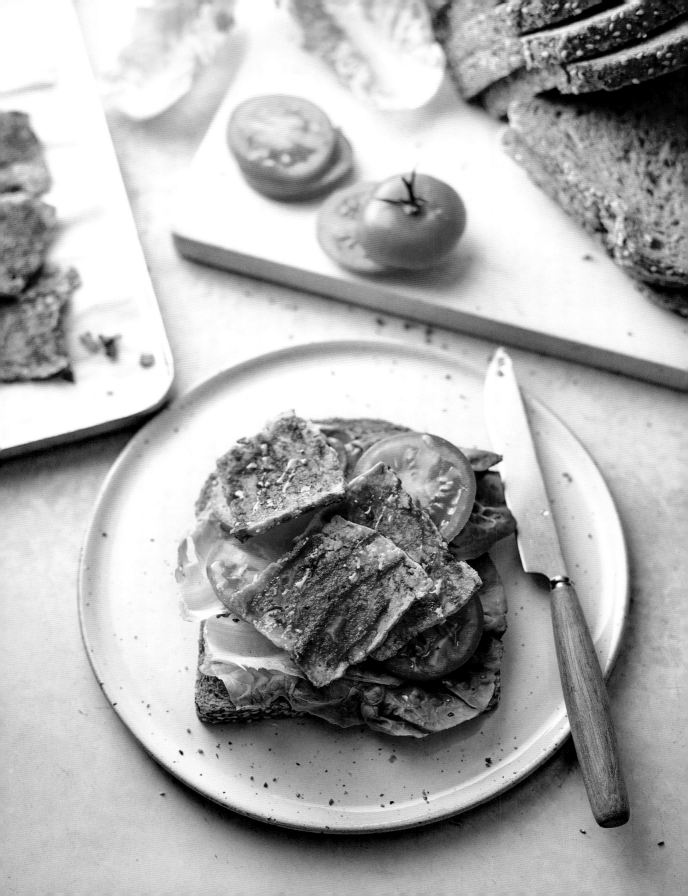

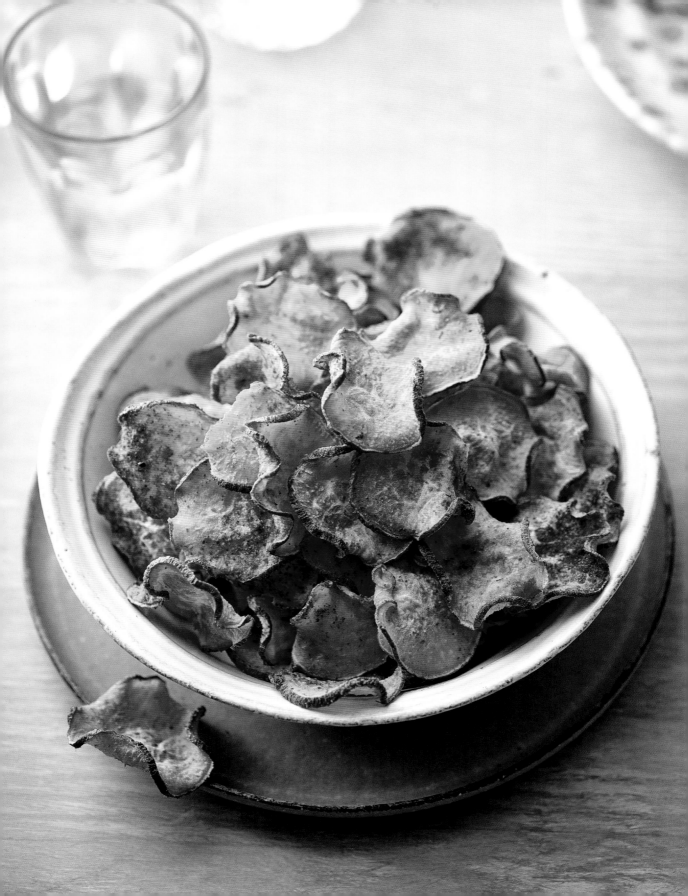

No-salt Vegetable Crisps

A low-salt homemade alternative to packet crisps. Sweet potatoes are rich in beta carotene and vitamin C, while beetroots are a good source of folate. Both have a natural sweetness.

SERVES 2–4 • 5 MINS • 25 MINS •

2 sweet potatoes, peeled,
   or 2 beetroot, trimmed
1 tbsp extra virgin olive oil
¼ tsp smoked paprika
Black pepper

1. Preheat the oven to 150°C/130°C fan/300°F/gas mark 2, line a couple of large baking trays with some baking paper.

2. Thinly slice the sweet potatoes or beetroot – you want the slices to be only a couple of millimetres thick. This is easiest with a mandolin, but you can use a sharp knife, or a vegetable peeler.

3. Toss the vegetables in a bowl with the olive oil, smoked paprika and a few grinds of black pepper. Mix together well, making sure each slice is evenly coated with oil.

4. Lay out the slices on the large, lined baking trays in a single layer. Bake for 20–25 minutes until dry – they will crisp up as they cool. Make sure you watch them carefully in the last 5 minutes of cooking, as they can burn quite easily.

5. Allow to cool then transfer to a bowl and eat.

TIP
You can also make super-simple crisps out of potato skin peelings. Just toss the peelings from 3 or 4 potatoes with 1 tablespoon of olive oil and bake at 180°C/160°C fan/350°F/gas mark 4 for 15–20 minutes, until lightly golden and slightly puffed.

Sesame & Rosemary Oatcakes

Even the 'healthy' oatcakes in a packet are high in salt, so these are a good low-salt or even no-salt version. You won't miss the salt here, as the seeds and rosemary add lots of flavour.

MAKES 30 CRACKERS • 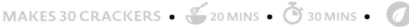 20 MINS • 30 MINS •

150g porridge oats
30g sesame seeds
1 tbsp finely chopped rosemary
Small pinch of salt (optional)
1 tbsp extra virgin olive oil
140g boiling water
Plain flour, for dusting

1. Preheat the oven to 180°C/160°C fan/350°F/gas mark 4 and line a large baking tray with baking paper.

2. Combine the oats, seeds, chopped rosemary, salt (if using) and oil in a large bowl. Pour over the boiling water, mix well, then leave for a few minutes so the oats can absorb the water.

3. Roll out the dough on a piece of baking paper until around 2–3mm thick. If you find the dough a bit sticky, dust lightly with plain flour when rolling. Cut the dough into circles using a round 6cm biscuit cutter (or a glass). The edges of the oatcakes may be a bit ragged – this is fine.

4. Transfer to the baking tray and bake for 25–30 minutes until crisp. Allow to cool on the tray then transfer to an airtight container to store for up to 2 weeks.

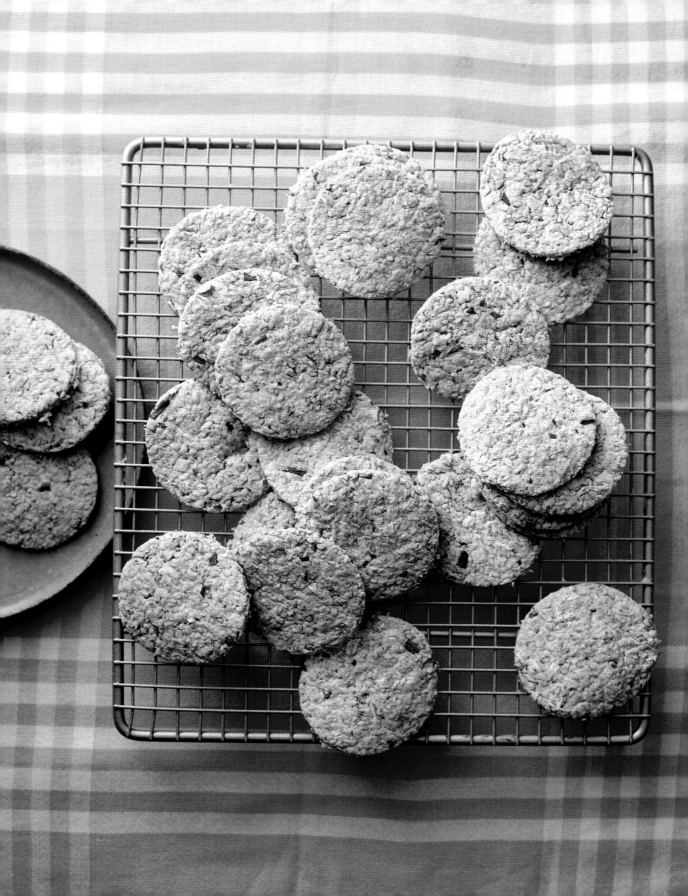

Courgette Hummus

This simple dip is made deliciously creamy through the courgette and white beans. The courgette adds hidden veg without impacting the flavours of the garlic and lemon.

SERVES 4 • 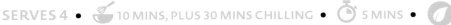 10 MINS, PLUS 30 MINS CHILLING • 5 MINS •

1 medium courgette

1 x 400g tin butterbeans or cannellini beans, drained and rinsed

3 tbsp lemon juice

2 tbsp extra virgin olive oil

2 tbsp tahini (optional)

1 garlic clove, crushed

Pinch of salt, to taste

1. Prick the courgette a few times with a fork or the sharp tip of a knife and place onto a baking tray. Place under a hot grill and cook until charred all over, turning occasionally – about 5 minutes. Set aside to cool completely.

2. Once cool enough to handle, peel off the skin and cut off the top of the stalk. Roughly chop the flesh and add to a food processor with the beans, lemon juice, oil, tahini (if using) and garlic. Blitz until smooth and creamy, then season with salt and blend again to combine.

3. Cover and chill for 30 minutes to allow the hummus to thicken, then serve.

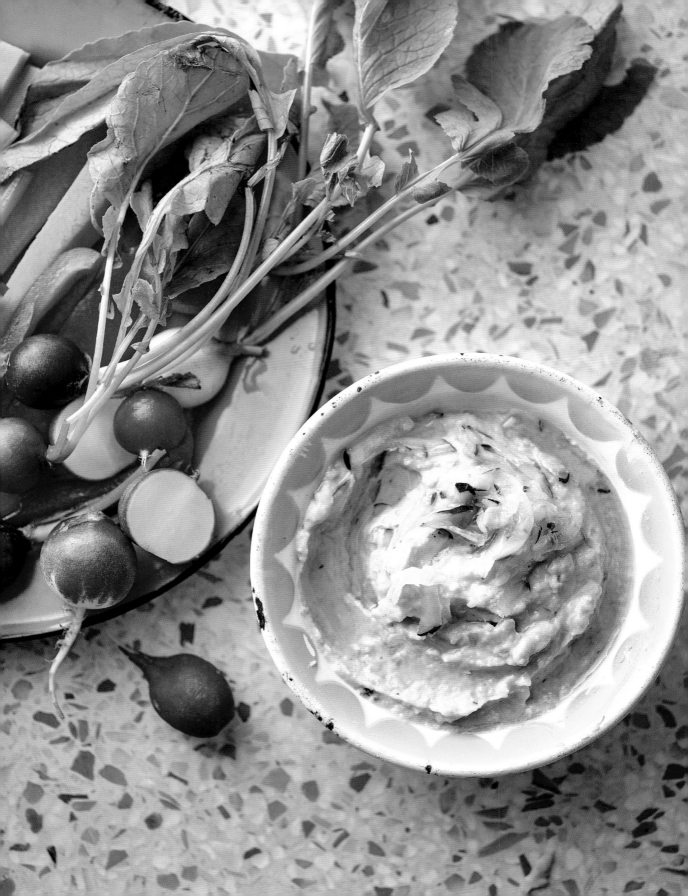

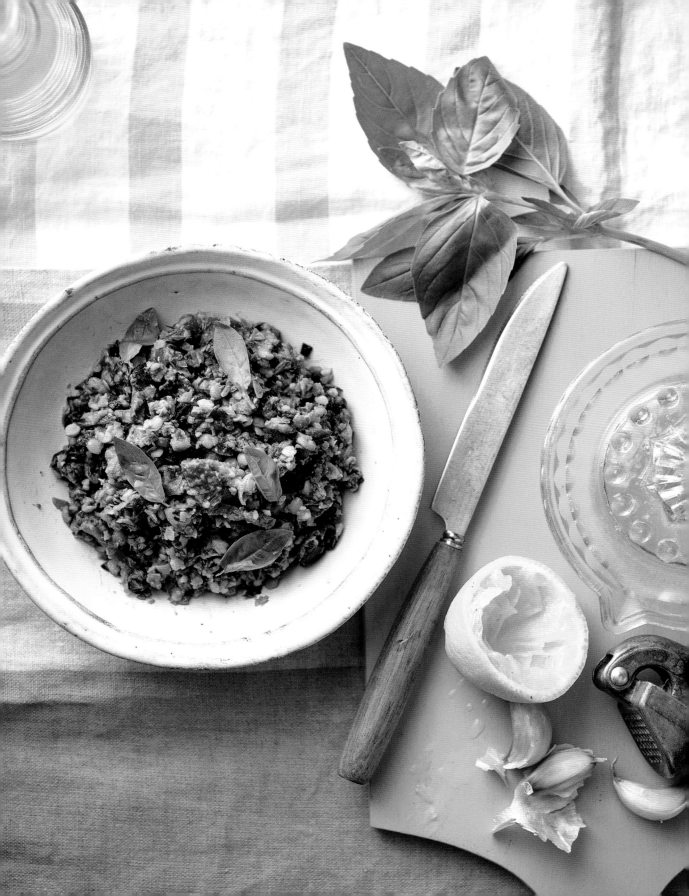

Olive & Lentil Tapenade

Used as a delicious topping for oatcakes (see page 92) or as crostini on toasted ciabatta. These make a really quick snack packed with protein and fibre. *(Pictured opposite.)*

SERVES 4 • 5 MINS • NONE •

30g fresh basil
160g pitted black olives
1 x 400g tin green lentils, drained
50g sun-dried tomatoes
Juice of 1 lemon
4 tbsp extra virgin olive oil
1 garlic clove, crushed

1. Add the basil to a food processor and blitz until well chopped. Add the olives, lentils, sun-dried tomatoes, lemon juice, oil and garlic. Pulse until you get a chunky purée, then transfer to a bowl and serve.

Chargrilled Vegetable Salsa

You don't notice the lack of salt here as the chargrilling adds so much smoky flavour to this vibrant and nutritious salsa. Serve with raw veg or toasted pita, or with grilled meat or chicken.

SERVES 4 • 10 MINS • 10 MINS •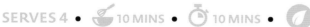

1 pepper
1 aubergine
40g walnuts
200g cherry tomatoes, halved
2 tbsp extra virgin olive oil
1 red onion, finely diced
Juice of ½ lemon
Handful of roughly chopped fresh basil, plus a few extra leaves for garnish

1. Place the pepper and aubergine over the flame of a gas hob, turning occasionally with tongs, until blackened all over – about 10 minutes. Alternatively, heat the grill, prick the aubergine and pepper with a knife and cook until blackened all over, turning occasionally.

2. Place the vegetables in a bowl, cover, then set aside. Once cool enough to handle, peel away the burnt skin. Remove the stems of the veg and seeds of the pepper.

3. Pulse the walnuts in a blender until roughly chopped. Add the aubergine, pepper and tomatoes and pulse to a rough salsa. Tip into a bowl, then stir in the oil, onion, lemon juice and basil. Garnish with some basil leaves.

Sesame Prawn Toasts

The perfect fakeaway – these homemade versions of the takeaway classic are grilled and lightly fried to reduce the fat content, are much lower in salt and use wholemeal bread for extra fibre.

MAKES 12 SLICES • 20 MINS • 🕐 10 MINS •

150g raw, peeled king prawns
(if frozen, defrosted)

2 garlic cloves, roughly chopped

2 spring onions, finely sliced, plus
extra for garnish

1 egg white

1 tsp sesame oil

½ tsp soy sauce

4 slices wholemeal bread,
crusts removed

2 tbsp vegetable oil

4 tbsp sesame seeds

FOR THE SWEET CHILLI SAUCE

2 tbsp water

1 tsp cornflour

2 red chillies, deseeded and
finely diced

2 tbsp orange juice

1 tbsp apple cider vinegar

1 tbsp honey

2 garlic cloves, crushed

1 tsp grated fresh ginger

1. Combine the prawns, garlic, spring onions, egg white, sesame oil and soy sauce in a food processor. Pulse to combine into a slightly chunky paste.

2. For the Sweet Chilli Sauce, combine the water and cornflour in a small pan until smooth. Stir in the chillies, orange juice, vinegar, honey, garlic and ginger. Cook over a medium heat until the mixture becomes translucent and thickens slightly. Remove from the heat and allow to cool.

3. Cut the slices of bread in half diagonally to get two triangles from each slice. Brush both sides with vegetable oil (using 1 tablespoon of the oil) and place on a baking tray. Pop under the grill and cook until golden, around 2 minutes. Flip and grill on the other side for another 2 minutes, until crisp and golden.

4. Place the sesame seeds into a wide dish. Spread the top of each triangle with the prawn mixture and dip the top into the sesame seeds to evenly coat.

5. Heat the remaining oil in a medium, non-stick pan. Add the toasts, prawn side down, and cook for 1–2 minutes on each side until golden on top and the prawns are cooked through. Remove to a plate, scatter over some sliced spring onions and serve with the Sweet Chilli Sauce in a bowl on the side.

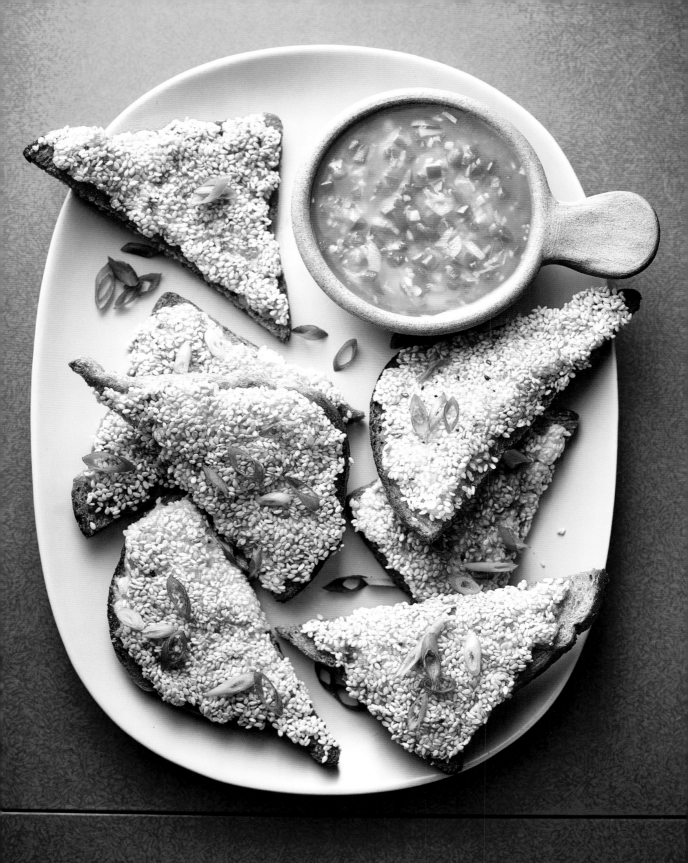

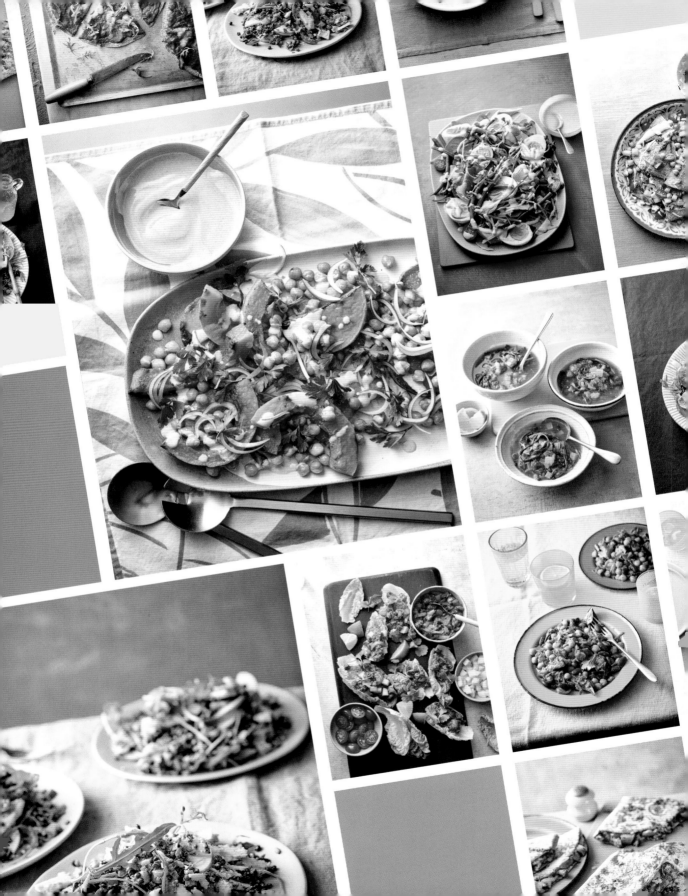

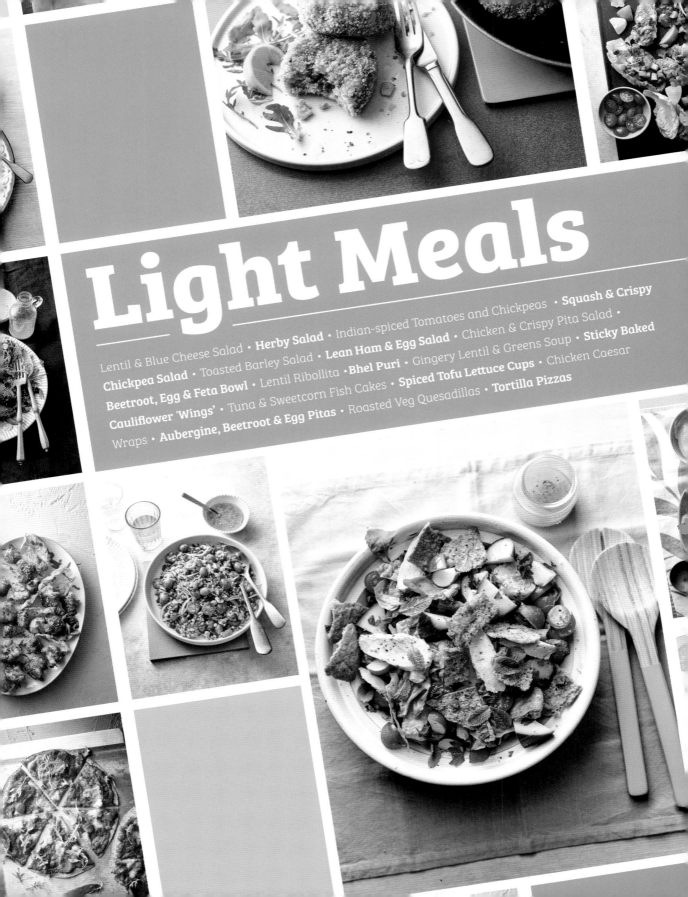

Light Meals

Lentil & Blue Cheese Salad · **Herby Salad** · Indian-spiced Tomatoes and Chickpeas · **Squash & Crispy Chickpea Salad** · Toasted Barley Salad · **Lean Ham & Egg Salad** · Chicken & Crispy Pita Salad · **Sticky Baked Beetroot, Egg & Feta Bowl** · Lentil Ribollita · **Bhel Puri** · Gingery Lentil & Greens Soup · Chicken Caesar **Cauliflower 'Wings'** · Tuna & Sweetcorn Fish Cakes · **Spiced Tofu Lettuce Cups** · Chicken Caesar Wraps · **Aubergine, Beetroot & Egg Pitas** · Roasted Veg Quesadillas · **Tortilla Pizzas**

Lentil & Blue Cheese Salad

Lentils add bulk, flavour and texture to a salad, and here the soft lentils are accompanied by crunchy apple and seeds, creamy blue cheese and a low-fat, probiotic dressing.

SERVES 4 • 15 MINS • 40 MINS •

1 tbsp olive oil

1 small red onion, finely diced

1 carrot, diced

250g dried Puy lentils or green lentils

1 bay leaf

90g rocket leaves

60g mixed seeds, such as sunflower, pumpkin, sesame, hemp, linseed

1 eating apple, cored and sliced thinly

100g blue cheese, crumbled

Handful of fresh parsley, roughly chopped

FOR THE DRESSING

4 tbsp natural yoghurt

1 tbsp lemon juice

1 tbsp extra virgin olive oil

1 tsp runny honey

1 garlic clove, crushed

Pinch of salt

1. Heat the olive oil in a medium pan over a medium heat. Add half of the onion and all of the carrot, then cook, stirring occasionally, until softened – around 10 minutes. Add the lentils and bay leaf to the pan and cover well with water. Bring to the boil over a high heat then turn down to simmer for 20–30 minutes, until the lentils are tender but not mushy.

2. Remove and discard the bay leaf, drain the contents of the pan, tip into a bowl and allow to cool.

3. Once cool, stir through the rocket, seeds, apple and remaining diced red onion.

4. Mix the dressing ingredients together and pour into the bowl with the salad, tossing everything together. Garnish with the crumbled blue cheese and parsley and serve.

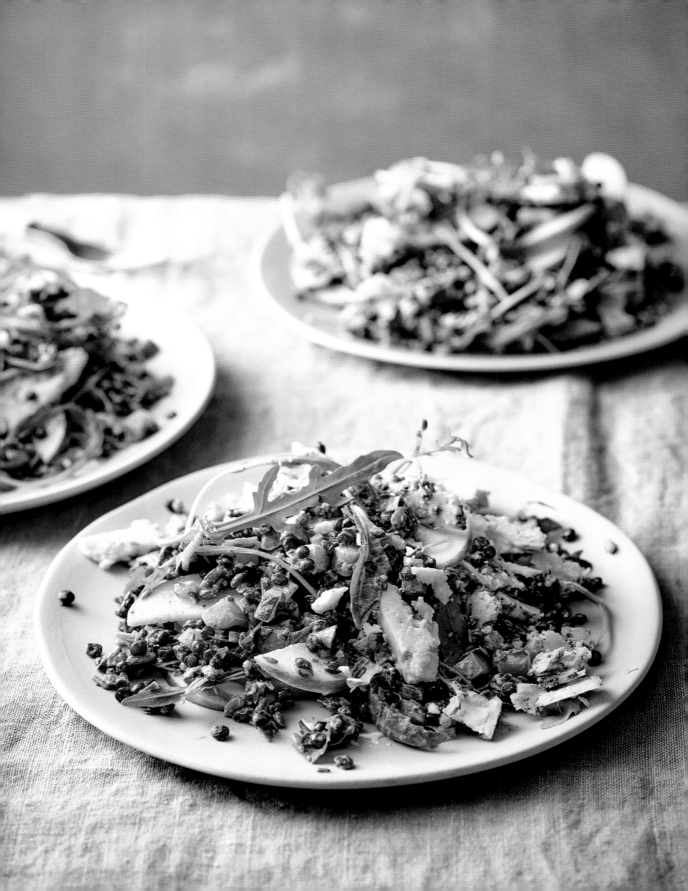

Herby Salad

A light and fresh-tasting salad that has plenty of crunch thanks to the radishes and sesame seeds. This needs no seasoning because it's full of the flavours of your favourite herbs.

SERVES 4 • 5 MINS • 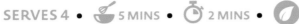 2 MINS •

120g mixed fresh herbs, such as dill, mint leaves, coriander, parsley, basil, chives

100g mixed salad leaves

100g radishes, thinly sliced

3 spring onions, thinly sliced

2 tbsp sesame seeds

FOR THE DRESSING

3 tbsp extra virgin olive oil

2 tbsp lemon juice

1 tsp finely grated lemon zest

2 tsp wholegrain mustard

Black pepper

1. Roughly chop the fresh herbs and add to a salad bowl with the salad leaves, radishes and spring onions. Toss together to combine.

2. Toast the sesame seeds in a small frying pan over a medium heat, stirring often, until golden and fragrant – keep an eye on these as they colour quickly and can burn. Tip into the salad bowl.

3. For the dressing, combine the olive oil, lemon juice and zest, mustard and a few good grinds of black pepper in a jar. Screw on the lid and shake to emulsify the mixture, then pour over the contents of the bowl. Toss the salad to coat with the dressing and serve.

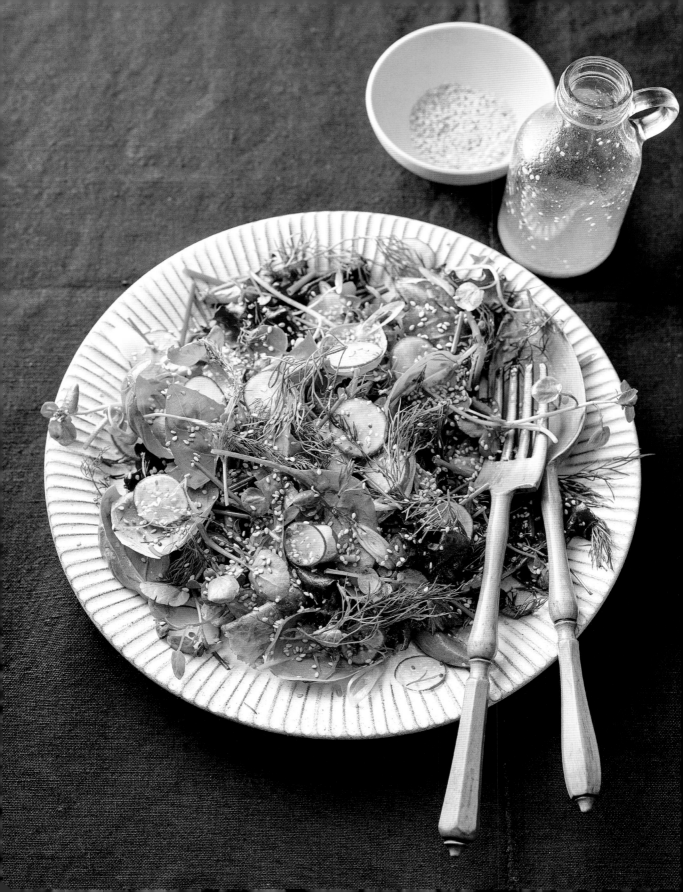

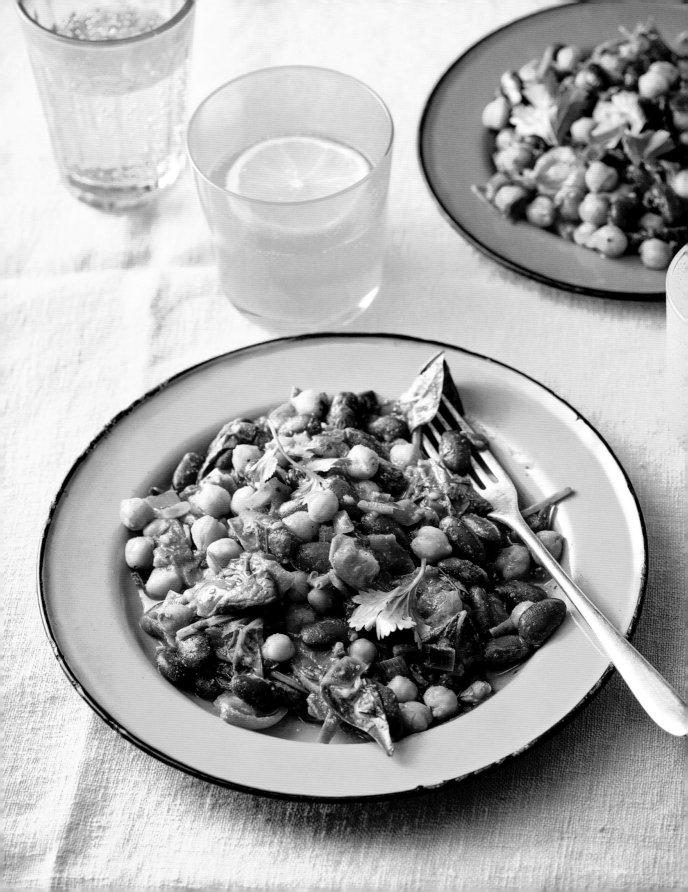

Indian-spiced Tomatoes and Chickpeas

Fresh, fibre-packed and filling, this is a treat for your gut! It's packed with protein and the cherry tomatoes and spinach add vital vitamins and minerals.

SERVES 4 • 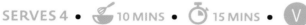 10 MINS • 15 MINS • V

1 tbsp vegetable oil

2 red onions, diced

6 tbsp tamarind sauce or 4 tbsp curry paste, such as tikka masala

1 x 400g tin chickpeas, drained and rinsed

1 x 400g tin kidney beans, drained and rinsed

250g cherry tomatoes, roughly chopped

100g baby spinach

Handful of fresh coriander, roughly chopped

Juice of 1 lemon

2 tsp mint sauce

Pinch of salt

1. Heat the oil in a medium, non-stick pan over a medium heat. Add the onions and cook until softened and turning golden, 5–7 minutes. Add the tamarind sauce or curry paste and cook for 1 more minute.

2. Add the chickpeas, kidney beans and cherry tomatoes to the pan. Cook until the tomatoes have softened, 3–4 minutes, then stir in the spinach and coriander until wilted. Remove from the heat, stir in the lemon juice and mint sauce, then season with salt, to taste.

Squash & Crispy Chickpea Salad

A lovely salad for an autumnal day – warming spices and the sweet flavours of roasted squash, with earthy chickpeas and vibrant herbs. A fresh and filling light meal.

SERVES 4 • 10 MINS • 45 MINS • V

1 butternut squash, peeled

1½ tbsp extra virgin olive oil

1 x 400g tin chickpeas, drained and rinsed

1 red onion, thinly sliced

Handful of fresh parsley, roughly chopped

Salt

FOR THE DRESSING

120g natural yoghurt

1 garlic clove, crushed

1 tsp smoked paprika

½ tsp chilli powder

1½ tbsp lemon juice

1 tsp runny honey

1. Preheat the oven to 200°C/180°C fan/400°F/gas mark 6.

2. Cut the neck of the squash in half then slice into 2cm thick semi-circles. Cut the base of the squash in half, scoop out and discard the seeds, then cut into 2cm thick arches. Toss with 1 tablespoon of the oil and a pinch of salt on a large tray. Roast for 45 minutes, flipping halfway through, until golden and soft.

3. Meanwhile, pat the chickpeas dry with a clean tea towel. Fry over a high heat in a small, non-stick pan with the remaining oil and a pinch of salt until starting to brown.

4. Place the squash wedges onto a platter and top with the chickpeas.

5. Mix the dressing ingredients in a small bowl, loosening with water. Drizzle over the salad and scatter with the sliced onion and parsley.

TIP
To make this into a more filling dish, serve with some cooked brown basmati rice and sprinkle over a handful of chopped, toasted walnuts or almonds.

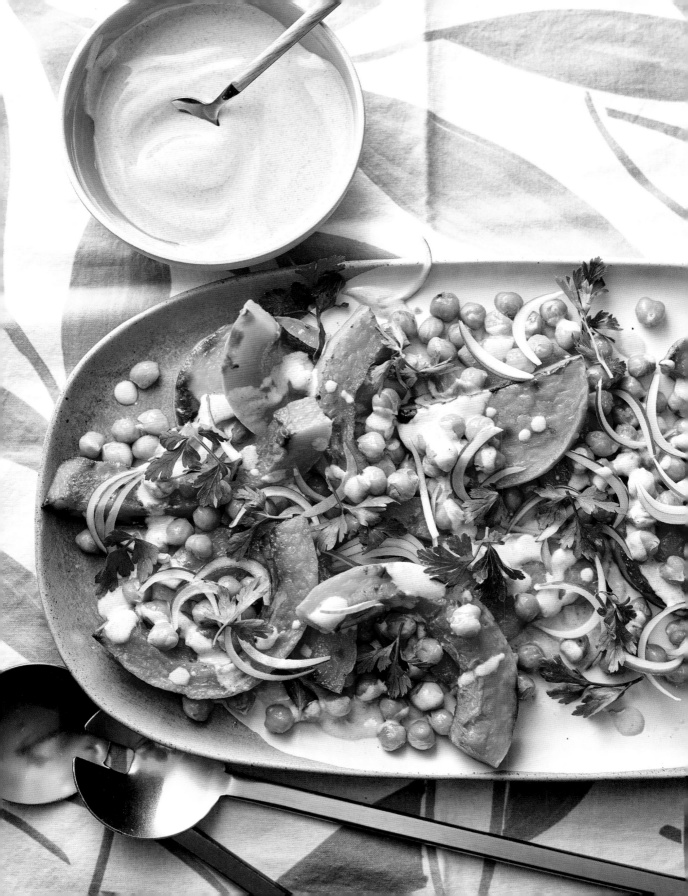

Toasted Barley Salad

Barley is a versatile wholegrain – perfect for salads, stews and to replace rice in risotto. It's packed with fibre but it's also low in fat, slowly releasing energy to avoid blood-sugar spikes.

SERVES 4 • 10 MINS • 1 HOUR •

1 tbsp extra virgin olive oil

175g pearl barley

Pinch of salt

100g sultanas or raisins

200g cherry tomatoes, halved

100g green olives, pitted

50g walnuts, roughly chopped

Handful of fresh parsley,
     roughly chopped

Handful of fresh coriander,
     roughly chopped

1 small red onion, thinly sliced

FOR THE DRESSING

3 tbsp extra virgin olive oil

Juice of 1 lemon

1 tbsp wholegrain mustard

Pinch of salt

A few good grinds of black pepper

1. Add the oil and pearl barley to a medium pan and set over a medium-high heat. Toast the barley, stirring constantly, until golden and fragrant – about 3 minutes. Remove from the heat so it can cool down a bit, then cover with water and add a pinch of salt. Return to a high heat, bring to a boil, turn down to simmer and cook for about 1 hour or until the barley is tender.

2. While the barley is cooking, mix the dressing ingredients together in a salad bowl. Stir in the sultanas or raisins, tomatoes and olives then set aside to marinate.

3. Once the barley is fully cooked, drain it and tip into the salad bowl. Fold in the walnuts, fresh herbs and red onions and serve.

TIP
Make ahead: assemble the salad but add the herbs at the last minute, as they will wilt. Store in the fridge in an airtight container for up to 3 days. Perfect for a lunchbox.

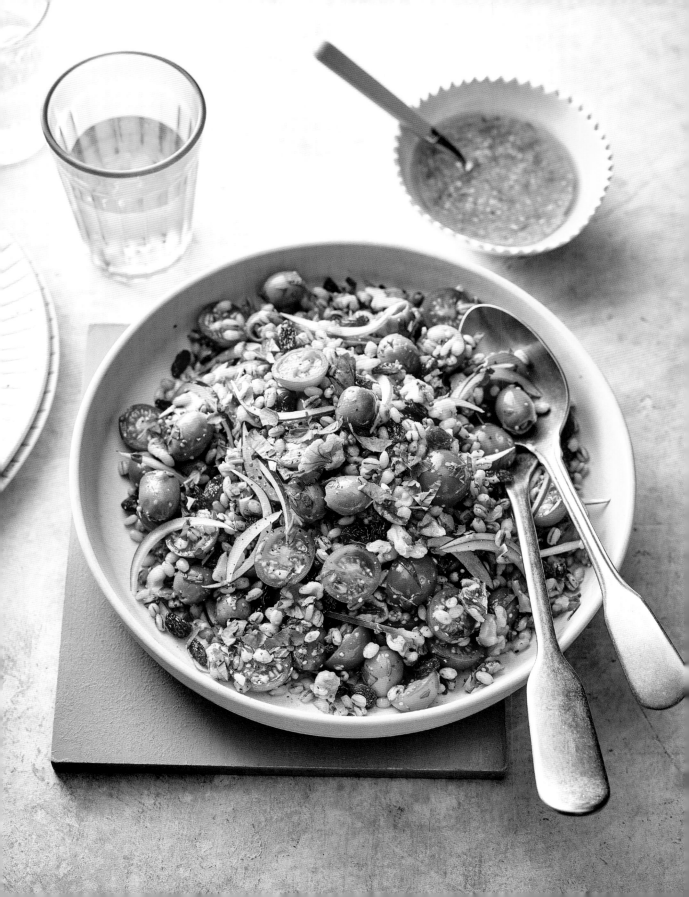

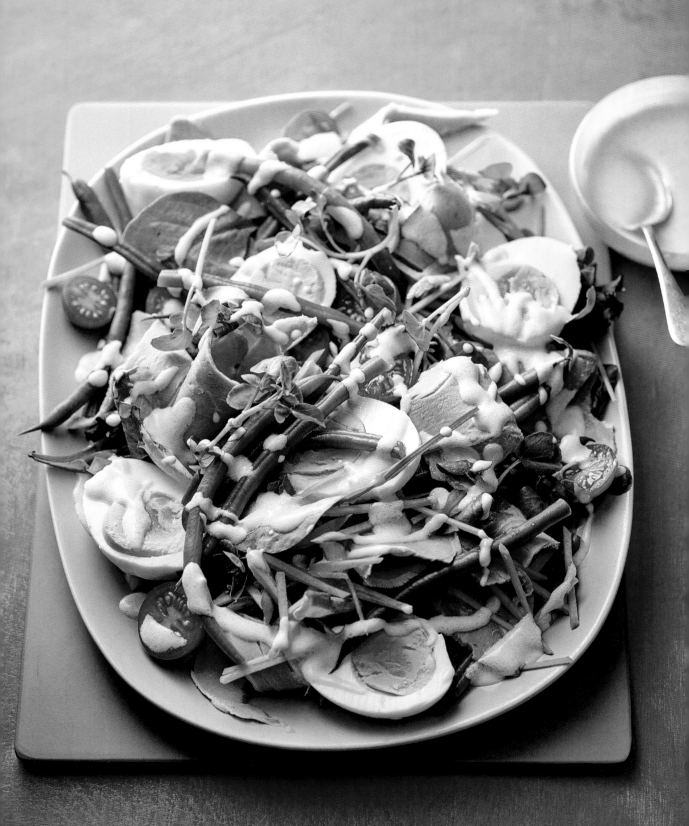

Lean Ham & Egg Salad

A lean and filling salad that makes a satisfying light meal. A rainbow of colours fills the plate, with lots of salad and veg. Protein from the ham and eggs will keep you going all day.

SERVES 4 • 10 MINS • 15 MINS •

4 eggs
200g green beans
250g cherry tomatoes, halved
200g bag mixed salad leaves
150g lean ham, torn
1 medium carrot, grated

FOR THE DRESSING
100g natural yoghurt
1 tbsp lemon juice
1 tbsp extra virgin olive oil
2 tsp Dijon mustard
1 garlic clove, crushed
Pinch of salt and ground black
    pepper

1. Bring a medium pan of water to the boil then turn the heat down to a gentle simmer. Carefully lower in the eggs then cook for 10 minutes. Remove the eggs from the pan with tongs or a slotted spoon to a bowl of cold water and set aside.

2. Keep the pan of water on the boil and add the green beans, cooking them for 4–5 minutes until tender, then drain and rinse under cold water.

3. Peel the cooled eggs then cut them in half. Add to a salad bowl with the green beans, cherry tomatoes, salad leaves, ham and the grated carrot.

4. Mix the dressing ingredients together in a small bowl then pour over the salad and toss together.

Chicken & Crispy Pita Salad

This Mediterranean-style salad is vibrant, fresh-tasting and crunchy, with chicken providing a lean source of protein and pita bread making higher-fibre croutons than standard bread.

SERVES 4 • 10 MINS • 10 MINS •

1 wholemeal pita bread

1 tbsp olive oil

½ tsp dried oregano

200g cherry tomatoes, halved

½ cucumber, thinly sliced

1 gem lettuce, leaves chopped

100g radishes, quartered

Handful of fresh parsley, roughly chopped

Handful of fresh mint leaves, roughly chopped, plus a few leaves for garnish

2 cooked chicken breasts, thinly sliced

FOR THE DRESSING

3 tbsp extra virgin olive oil

2 tbsp lemon juice

1 garlic clove, crushed

¼ tsp ground cumin

Pinch of salt

1. Preheat the oven to 200°C/180°C fan/400°F/gas mark 6.

2. Rip the pita bread into bite-sized pieces then toss with the olive oil and oregano on a large baking tray, spreading them out into a single layer. Bake for 6–10 minutes, until golden and crisp.

3. Combine the tomatoes, cucumber, lettuce, radishes, parsley, mint, chicken and crispy pita chips in a salad bowl and toss together.

4. Mix the dressing ingredients together in a jar and shake to combine. Pour over the salad and toss to coat, then serve immediately, scattered with a few mint leaves.

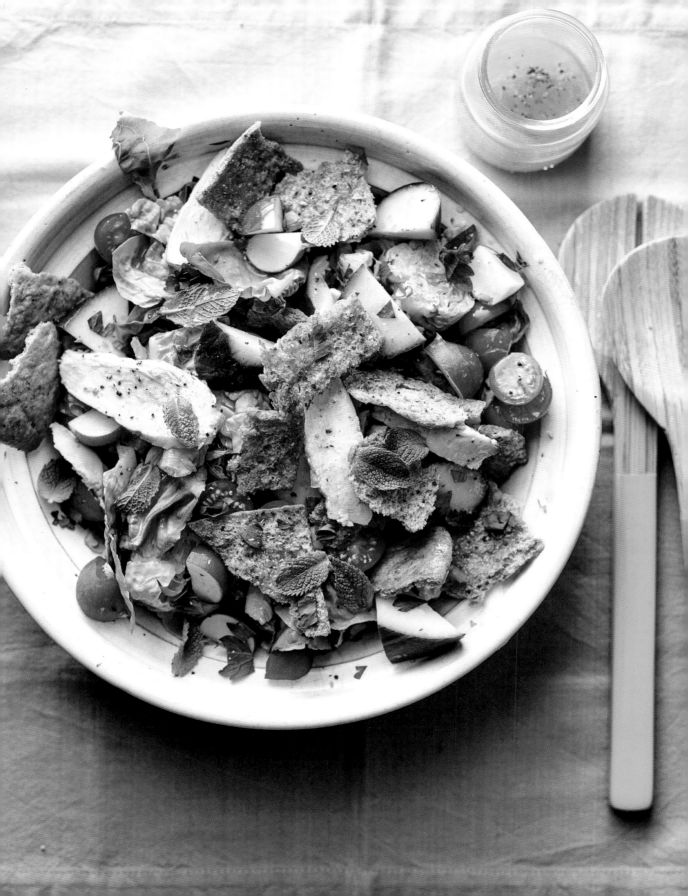

Beetroot, Egg & Feta Bowl

Bursting with goodness, this colourful salad is full of textures and flavours, from earthy beetroot to crunchy pumpkin seeds and soft feta. A great bowl of fibre, folate and protein.

SERVES 4 • 15 MINS • 1 HOUR • ⓥ

500g beetroot

4 eggs

2 tbsp pumpkin seeds

80g feta cheese, cubed

90g rocket leaves

Handful of fresh mint leaves, roughly chopped

FOR THE DRESSING

½ shallot, finely diced

2 tbsp balsamic vinegar

2 tbsp extra virgin olive oil

Pinch of salt

1. Preheat the oven to 200°C/180°C fan/400°F/gas mark 6.

2. Trim the stems off the beetroot and wrap in a piece of foil. Place onto a baking tray and roast for 45 minutes–1 hour, until tender.

3. Meanwhile, bring a small pan of water to the boil then turn the heat down to low. Gently lower in the eggs and cook for either 6 minutes (for soft-boiled) or 10 minutes (for hard-boiled). Drain the eggs then cover with cold water.

4. Heat the pumpkin seeds in a small pan over a high heat until they start to pop. Remove from the heat and tip into a salad bowl.

5. Rub the skins off the cooked beets under running water then dice them into 1cm chunks. Add to the salad bowl with the feta, rocket and mint.

6. Combine the dressing ingredients in a jar and shake to emulsify, then pour over the salad, toss to coat and divide between 4 plates. Peel the eggs and slice into quarters then place on top of each salad.

Lentil Ribollita

A simple soup that is made with humble veg and is full of flavour. It's a deliciously satisfying soup, thanks to the lentils and cannellini beans, which pack a fibre and protein punch.

SERVES 4 • 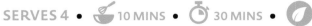 10 MINS • 30 MINS •

2 tbsp extra virgin olive oil

2 red onions

2 carrots

2 celery sticks

Pinch of salt

200g cherry tomatoes, halved

3 garlic cloves, crushed

1 tbsp finely chopped rosemary leaves

1.5 litres veg stock (2 cubes)

1 x 400g tin cannellini beans

100g dried red lentils

100g chopped kale

2 slices stale, crusty bread, torn into chunks

1. Heat the olive oil in a large pan over a medium heat. Add the onions, carrots, celery and a pinch of salt. Cook until starting to soften, around 5 minutes, then stir in the tomatoes, garlic and rosemary. Cook until the tomatoes are soft, another 5 minutes, then pour in the stock. Tip in the tin of cannellini beans – along with the liquid from the tin – and the red lentils.

2. Bring to the boil, add the kale and torn bread, turn down to simmer and cook for 20 minutes until the lentils are soft.

Bhel Puri

This easy to prep and very moreish salad is a feast for your gut. Prebiotic chickpeas and red onion work with probiotic natural yoghurt to feed good gut bacteria and keep them healthy.

SERVES 4 • 15 MINS • 7 MINS • (V)

2 wholemeal tortillas

1 tbsp olive oil

1 x 400g tin chickpeas, drained and rinsed

250g cherry tomatoes, quartered

1 small red onion, finely diced

4 tbsp natural yoghurt

½ ripe mango, peeled and diced, or 1 eating apple, diced

20g wholegrain puffed rice cereal (optional)

FOR THE CORIANDER CHUTNEY

15g fresh coriander, roughly chopped

10g fresh mint leaves (or more coriander)

2 tbsp lemon juice

1 garlic clove, peeled

1 green chilli, seeds removed

6g grated fresh ginger

Pinch of salt

1. Blitz all the chutney ingredients together in a blender until you get a mostly smooth paste. Set aside.

2. Use a pair of scissors to cut the tortillas into roughly 5cm wide triangles. Toss with the olive oil on a large baking tray and spread out in a single layer. Bake for 5–7 minutes until just turning golden. They'll crisp up as they cool.

3. Lay half of the tortilla chips onto a serving plate. Top with half of the chickpeas, half of the tomatoes and half of the onion. Drizzle with half the yoghurt and half the chutney.

4. Repeat the layering, using the remaining tortilla chips, chickpeas, tomatoes, onion, yoghurt and chutney.

5. Finally, scatter over the mango and puffed rice cereal, if using. Serve immediately.

TIPS
You can make extra chutney and freeze it for up to 3 months.

Swap the mango for the seeds of ½ pomegranate.

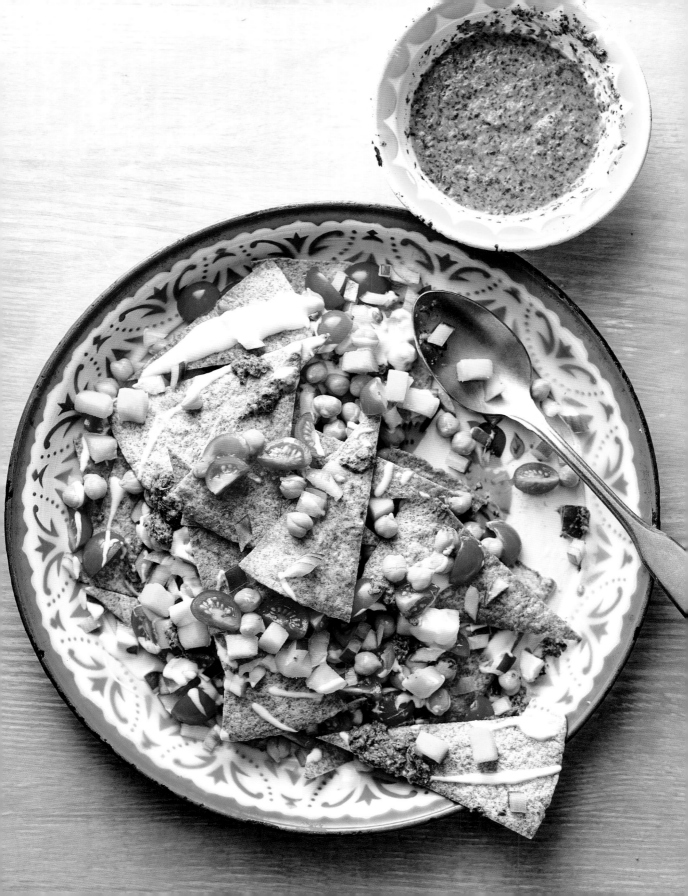

Gingery Lentil & Greens Soup

The bulk of this delicious and warming soup is provided by cheap, everyday vegetables that provide a rainbow of colour and a variety of textures, flavours and nutrients.

SERVES 4 • 10 MINS • 30 MINS •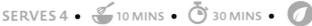

2 tbsp extra virgin olive oil

2 onions, diced

2 carrots, diced

2 celery sticks, diced

Pinch of salt

4 garlic cloves, crushed

2 tsp cumin seeds

2 tsp grated fresh ginger

1 x 400g tin chopped tomatoes

1 litre water

1 vegetable stock cube

1 x 250g pouch cooked Puy lentils, or 1 x 400g tin cooked green lentils, drained and rinsed

200g baby spinach

4 lemon wedges, to serve

1. Heat the oil in a medium pan over a medium heat. Add the onions, carrots, celery and a pinch of salt. Cook for 10 minutes, stirring occasionally, until the veg have softened.

2. Add the garlic, cumin seeds and ginger and cook for 1 minute more. Pour in the chopped tomatoes and water then crumble in the stock cube and add the lentils. Bring to the boil then turn down to simmer and cook for 15–20 minutes to allow the flavours to develop.

3. Stir in the baby spinach until wilted, divide between 4 bowls and serve with lemon wedges for squeezing.

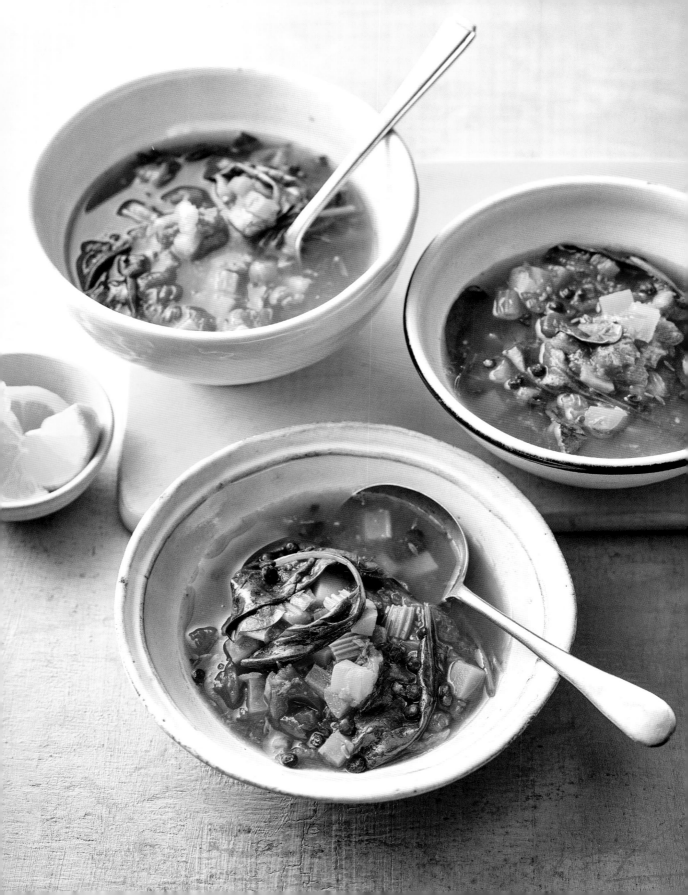

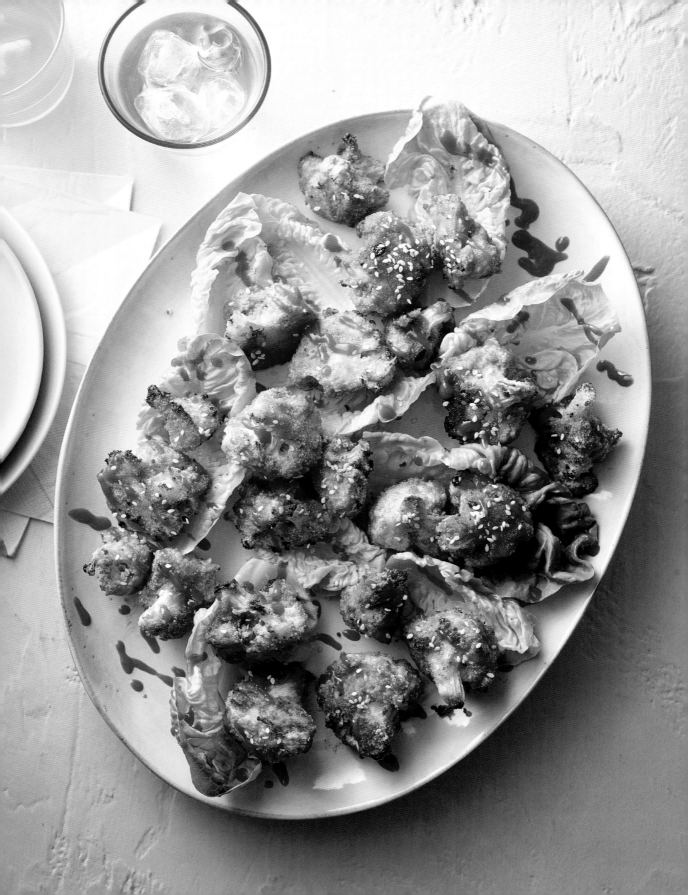

Sticky Baked Cauliflower 'Wings'

Cauliflower florets make a clever veggie swap for chicken wings; they are lower in fat, but have a delicious crunchy texture even when baked, and the sticky glaze lifts the overall flavours.

SERVES 4 • 25 MINS • 50 MINS •

1 tbsp vegetable oil

50g wholemeal plain flour

1 tbsp cornflour

80g water

650g (1 medium) cauliflower, separated into florets

2 tbsp golden breadcrumbs

FOR THE STICKY GLAZE

2 tbsp soy sauce

1 tbsp runny honey

1 tsp apple cider vinegar

1 tsp sriracha

1 tsp garlic granules

1 tsp sesame oil

TO SERVE

2 gem lettuce, outer leaves separated

1 tbsp sesame seeds

1. Preheat the oven to 200°C/180°C fan/400°F/gas mark 6 and line a large, rimmed baking tray with baking paper. Brush half of the oil over the baking paper and set side.

2. In a large bowl mix the flour, cornflour and water together to get a thin batter. Add the cauliflower florets and toss to coat them with the batter. Sprinkle the breadcrumbs into the batter mix and stir them in. Lay the coated florets out on the greased tray and drizzle with the remaining vegetable oil. Bake for 20–30 minutes, or until the florets have softened.

3. Meanwhile, combine the sticky glaze ingredients in a small bowl and stir until smooth.

4. Once the florets are out of the oven, tip them into a large bowl and pour over the glaze. Toss to coat fully with the glaze then spread the florets out on the tray again. Bake for a further 20 minutes until the glaze is sticky and the florets are slightly crisp.

5. Serve the cauliflower warm in lettuce leaf 'cups', sprinkled with sesame seeds.

Tuna & Sweetcorn Fish Cakes

Using mostly storecupboard ingredients these fish cakes are the perfect light meal in a hurry and are super cheap to make, too. Tuna contains omega 3 even when bought in tins.

SERVES 4 • 20 MINS • 30 MINS •

350g potatoes, peeled and cut into 3cm chunks

1 x 400g tin haricot beans or cannellini beans, drained

1 x 150g (drained weight) tuna packed in olive oil

150g frozen sweetcorn, defrosted

50g sun-dried tomatoes, roughly chopped

Handful of fresh basil, parsley or chives, roughly chopped

1 egg, beaten

100g dried breadcrumbs, preferably wholemeal

2–3 tbsp olive oil

Salt and freshly ground black pepper

Lemon wedges, to serve

TIP
These freeze well, so make in batches and freeze before cooking. Defrost before frying.

1. Place the potatoes in a medium pan and cover with water. Bring to the boil then turn the heat down to a simmer and cook for 10–15 minutes until very soft. Drain, return to the pan and mash until smooth. Add the drained beans and partially mash them in with a potato masher.

2. Flake the drained tuna into the mash. Add the sweetcorn, sun-dried tomatoes and chopped herbs. Mix everything together and season with salt and black pepper, to taste. Pour in half of the beaten egg and stir together. Divide the mixture into 8 balls and flatten into patties.

3. Loosen the remaining beaten egg with a splash of water in a wide bowl. Place the breadcrumbs in another bowl. Dip each patty into the egg mix, letting the excess drip off, then dredge in the breadcrumbs to evenly coat both sides.

4. Heat 1 tablespoon of the oil in a medium, non-stick frying pan. Add 3–4 fish cakes at a time and fry over a medium heat for 2–3 minutes on each side until golden. Set aside and keep warm while you cook the remaining fish cakes. Serve with lemon wedges for squeezing over.

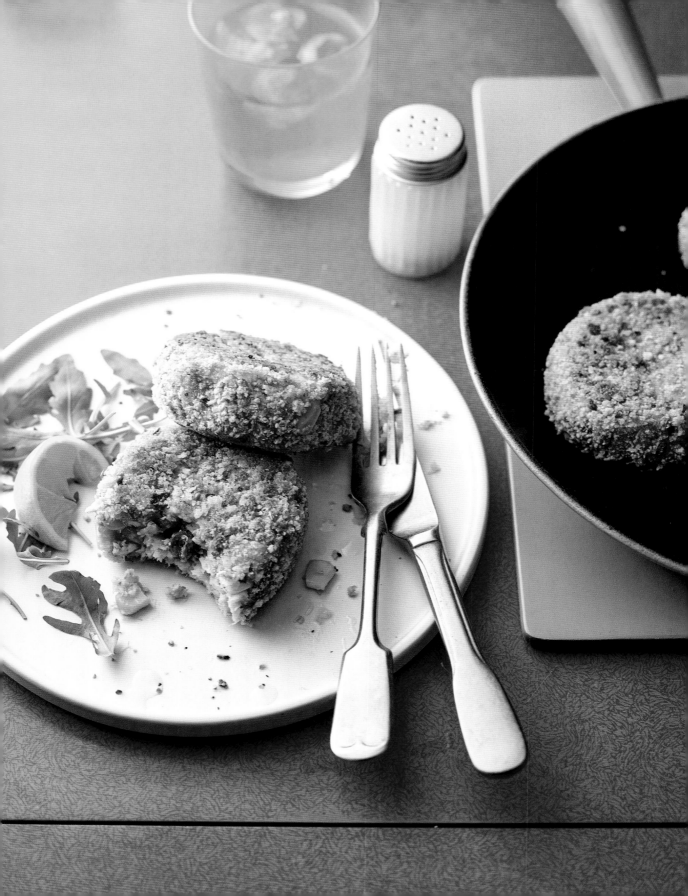

Spiced Tofu Lettuce Cups

Crumbled tofu makes a brilliant plant-based alternative to mince, while still being high in protein and low in fat, and is perked up with herbs, spices and fresh fruit for more flavour.

SERVES 4 • 15 MINS, PLUS 30 MINS RESTING • 12 MINS •

280g firm tofu

1 tbsp soy sauce

1 tbsp extra virgin olive oil

2 onions, diced

300g frozen sliced peppers

2 tbsp tomato purée

2 tsp ground cumin

2 tsp smoked paprika

1 tsp garlic granules

½ tsp ground cinnamon

3 gem lettuce, outer leaves separated and washed

1 mango, diced, or 2 eating apples (preferably Jazz or Pink Ladies), cored and diced

150g cherry tomatoes, halved

Handful of fresh coriander

1 lime, quartered, to serve

1. Drain the tofu then wrap in a clean tea towel and place on a board. Place another board on top and weigh it down with a few books. Set aside for 30 minutes to allow the excess water to be gently removed from the tofu. Unwrap and crumble the tofu into a bowl. Stir in the soy sauce and set aside.

2. Heat the oil in a large, non-stick frying pan over a medium-low heat. Add the onions and cook until starting to soften, around 5 minutes. Add the frozen peppers and turn the heat up to medium, then cook until the peppers and onions are turning golden, another 5 minutes. Add the crumbled tofu and stir until warmed through. Mix in the tomato purée, cumin, smoked paprika, garlic and cinnamon for 1 minute then remove from the heat.

3. Scoop the tofu mixture into the gem lettuce 'cups', with the mango (or apple), tomatoes and coriander and serve with the lime quarters.

TIP
The varieties of apple listed here are sweeter than others, so they work well as a replacement for mango. Or you can also choose your favourite apple variety.

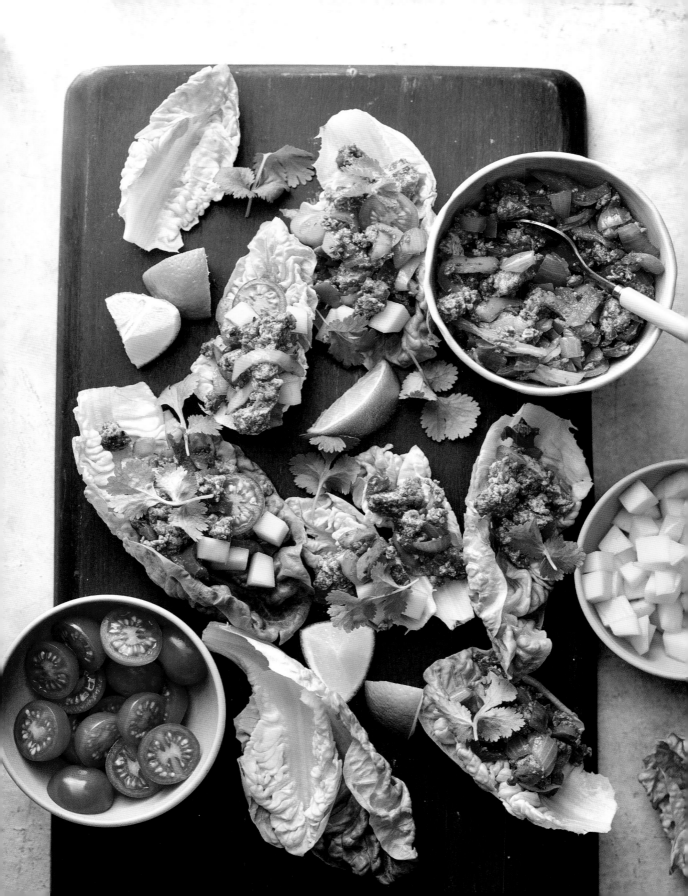

Chicken Caesar Wraps

A more filling version of the classic salad, using wholemeal wraps rather than fried croutons making it lower in fat. A yoghurt-based dressing replaces the high-fat Caesar dressing.

SERVES 4 • 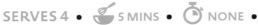 5 MINS • NONE •

4 wholemeal tortillas

2 heads little gem lettuce, chopped

2 cooked skinless chicken breasts, thinly sliced

200g tomatoes, diced

FOR THE DRESSING

4 anchovies

70g natural yoghurt

50g hummus

2 tbsp finely grated Parmesan cheese

1 tbsp extra virgin olive oil

1 tbsp lemon juice

1 tsp Dijon mustard

1. Start with the dressing. Mash the anchovies with the back of a fork into a paste then scrape into a bowl. Mix in the remaining dressing ingredients.

2. Lay out the tortillas and top with the chopped lettuce, sliced chicken and diced tomatoes. Drizzle the dressing over the fillings.

3. Fold in the sides of the tortilla then roll up tightly into a log, slice in half and serve.

TIPS

If you don't have hummus, replace it with 50g natural yoghurt and add 1 small, crushed garlic clove to the dressing.

Make ahead: make the dressing and store in a clean jar for up to 3 days in the fridge.

Aubergine, Beetroot & Egg Pitas

High-fibre wraps that are colourful, tasty and full of flavour, with soft and golden fried aubergine, tangy homemade beetroot pickle and creamy hummus.

SERVES 4 • 15 MINS • 20 MINS • Ⓥ

2 small beetroot, peeled and coarsely grated

1 small red onion, thinly sliced

Juice of 1 lemon

2 aubergines, sliced into 1cm thick coins

1 tbsp olive oil

4 large eggs

4 tbsp hummus

4 wholemeal pita breads, halved

Handful of parsley, chopped

Salt and freshly ground black pepper

1. Place the grated beetroot and sliced onion into a small bowl and mix in the lemon juice with a pinch of salt.

2. Lay the aubergine slices on a board and sprinkle with salt. Set aside for 5 minutes then blot the excess water off the aubergine slices with kitchen paper.

3. Heat a large non-stick pan over a high heat. Once hot, drizzle 1 tablespoon of olive oil into the pan and fry the aubergines for 5 minutes until browned underneath, then flip and cook for another 5 minutes. Repeat until all the aubergine slices are cooked.

4. Meanwhile, bring a small pan of water to the boil, turn down to a gentle simmer and slowly lower in the eggs. Cook for 6 minutes then remove the eggs from the water to a bowl of cold water. Once cool enough to handle, peel off the shells, cut the eggs in half and set aside.

5. Spread the hummus into each of the pita halves and fill with some of the beetroot-onion mixture (leaving behind the juice in the bowl), the fried aubergine slices and the halved eggs. Sprinkle with the parsley and serve.

TIPS

If you prefer a hard-boiled egg, boil the eggs for 8–10 minutes.

You can use homemade hummus here or the courgette hummus on page 94.

Roasted Veg Quesadillas

A Mexican-inspired snack packed with fibre and vitamins from sweet potatoes, peppers, beans and wholemeal wraps. Using less cheese keeps the flavour but makes the dish lower in fat.

SERVES 4 • 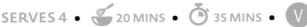 20 MINS • 35 MINS • V

500g sweet potatoes, peeled and cut into 2cm chunks

2 peppers, deseeded and cut into thin strips

1 tbsp extra virgin olive oil

1 x 400g tin kidney beans

1½ tsp ground cumin

½ tsp cayenne pepper

1 tbsp apple cider vinegar

6 large wholemeal tortillas

100g mature Cheddar cheese

Salt

1. Preheat the oven to 220°C/200°C fan/425°F/gas mark 7.

2. Toss the sweet potatoes and peppers with the oil and a pinch of salt on a large baking tray and roast for 20 minutes until softened.

3. Drain the kidney beans, reserving 2 tablespoons of the liquid from the tin, and tip the beans into a bowl. Mash with a potato masher to get a coarse paste then stir in the reserved bean liquid, the cumin, cayenne and vinegar. Season with a pinch of salt and set aside.

4. Take one tortilla and spread a bit of the kidney bean mash over one half of it. Scatter on some of the roast veg and top with a sprinkle of cheese. Fold in half and place into a hot frying pan over a high heat. Cook for 3–4 minutes until the underside is golden then flip and cook for a further 3–4 minutes until the other side is golden. Remove to a board and slice in half to get two wedges.

5. Fill and cook the remaining tortillas in the same fashion.

TIPS

Make ahead: roast the veg and mash the beans and store in airtight containers in the fridge for up to 5 days or the freezer for up to 3 months.

Use any veg you have to hand – cauliflower or broccoli florets, squash or carrots.

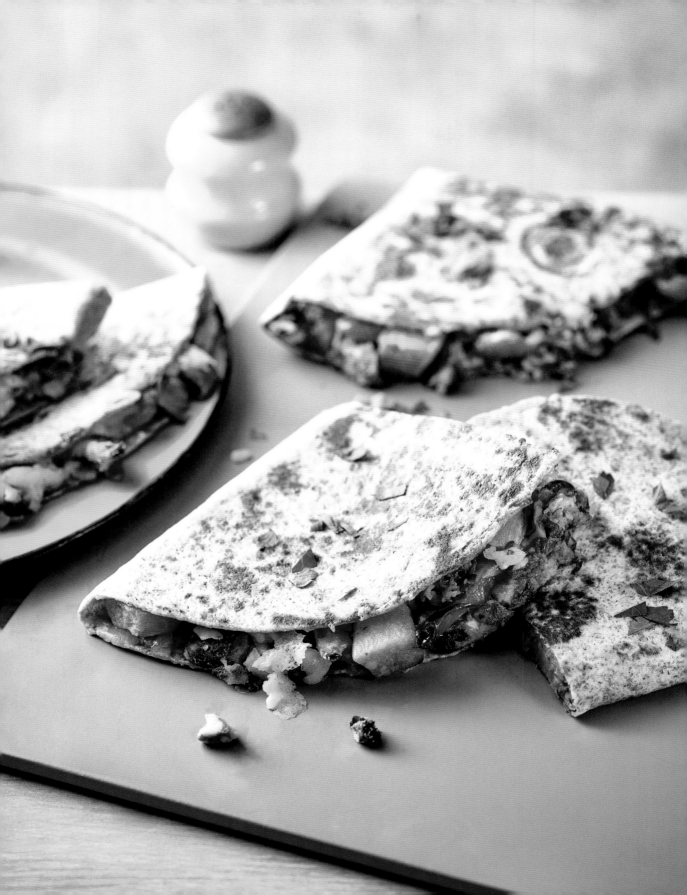

Tortilla Pizzas

A simple option for fakeaway Friday! Wholemeal pittas make a higher-fibre, lower-fat alternative to traditional pizza dough, and are much quicker to assemble.

SERVES 4 • 15 MINS • 30 MINS •

4 large wholemeal or seeded tortillas

125g ball mozzarella cheese, roughly chopped

A few handfuls of rocket leaves

FOR THE HIDDEN VEG TOMATO SAUCE

1 tbsp olive oil

2 onions, diced

2 peppers, deseeded and diced

1 courgette, finely grated

1 carrot, finely grated

1 x 200g tube tomato purée

1 x 400g tin chopped tomatoes

250ml water

1 tbsp balsamic vinegar

1 tbsp finely chopped rosemary leaves

2 tsp dried oregano

Pinch of salt

1. First make the tomato sauce. Heat the oil in a large pan over a medium heat. Add the onion and peppers then cook until they start to brown, 5–7 minutes. Stir in the grated courgette, carrot, tomato purée, chopped tomatoes, water, balsamic, rosemary and oregano and a pinch of salt. Simmer for 10 minutes over a low heat, stirring occasionally, to allow the sauce to thicken. Remove from the heat and, if you like, give it a quick blitz with a hand blender to make a smoother sauce.

2. Preheat the oven to 200°C/180°C fan/400°F/gas mark 6.

3. Lay a couple of tortillas out on a large baking tray. Spread 3 tablespoons (80g) of sauce over each tortilla, leaving a slight border uncovered. Top with a quarter of the cheese then cook in the oven for 5–7 minutes until the cheese has melted. Top with the rocket and cut each pizza into wedges. Repeat with the remaining wraps.

TIPS

The sauce is also great for serving with pasta.

Make a bigger batch of sauce and freeze in small sandwich bags, putting 320g (4 x 80g) into each. If you flatten these when you freeze them, they will defrost quicker!

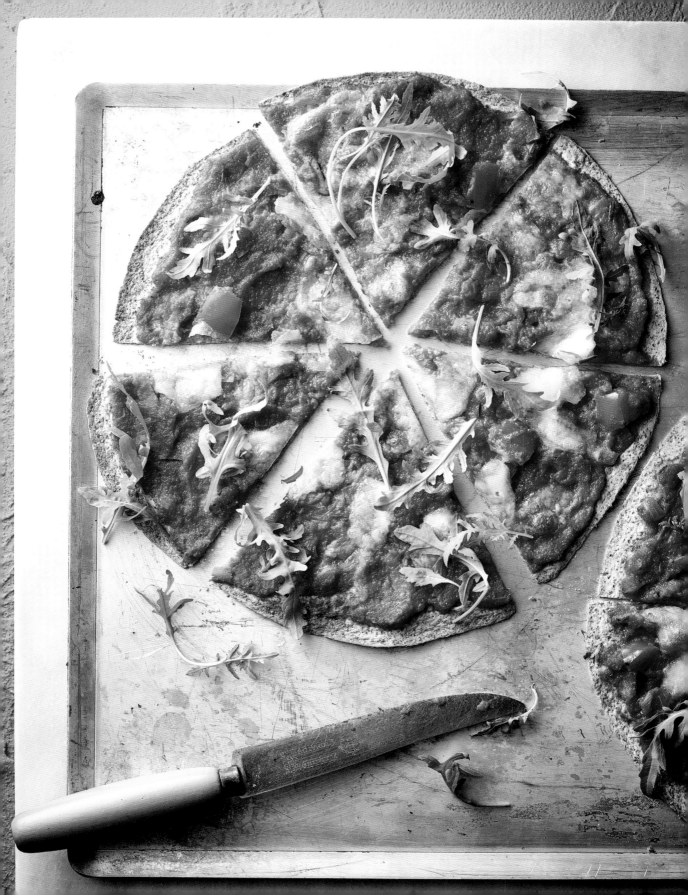

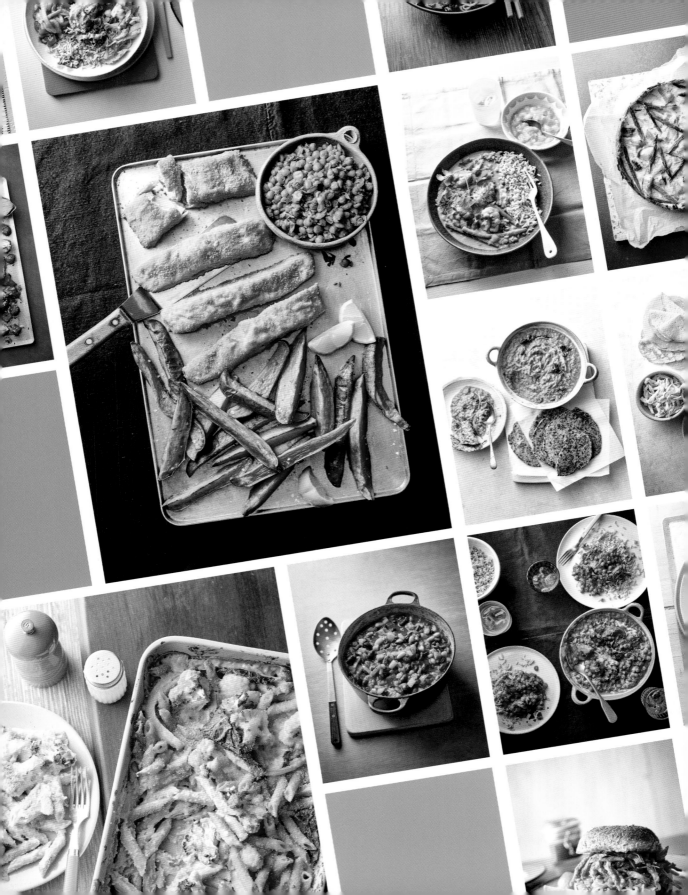

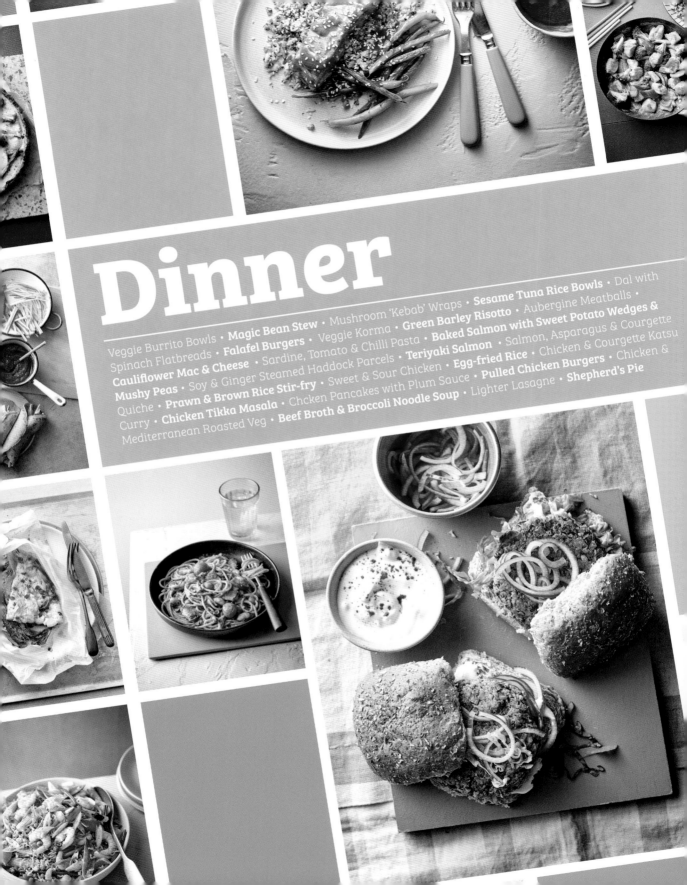

Dinner

Veggie Burrito Bowls • **Magic Bean Stew** • Mushroom 'Kebab' Wraps • **Sesame Tuna Rice Bowls** • Dal with Spinach Flatbreads • **Falafel Burgers** • Veggie Korma • **Green Barley Risotto** • Aubergine Meatballs • **Cauliflower Mac & Cheese** • Sardine, Tomato & Chilli Pasta • **Baked Salmon with Sweet Potato Wedges & Mushy Peas** • Soy & Ginger Steamed Haddock Parcels • **Teriyaki Salmon** • Salmon, Asparagus & Courgette Quiche • **Prawn & Brown Rice Stir-fry** • Sweet & Sour Chicken • **Egg-fried Rice** • Chicken & Courgette Katsu Curry • **Chicken Tikka Masala** • Chcken Pancakes with Plum Sauce • Lighter Lasagne • **Shepherd's Pie** • Mediterranean Roasted Veg • **Beef Broth & Broccoli Noodle Soup** • Chicken & Pulled Chicken Burgers • Chicken &

Veggie Burrito Bowls

This quick and easy supper contains all the essential amino acids in one bowl, so it's perfect for vegetarians. The rainbow of vegetables provides a big hit of phytonutrients, too.

SERVES 4 • 15 MINS • 15 MINS •

2 tbsp extra virgin olive oil

2 onions, sliced

400g frozen sliced peppers

2 x 400g tins black beans

1 x 400g tin chopped tomatoes

2 tsp ground cumin

2 tsp smoked paprika

1 tsp ground coriander

500g cooked brown basmati rice

1 avocado, peeled, stoned and mashed

1 gem lettuce, finely shredded

Hot sauce, to serve

FOR THE SALSA

120g cherry tomatoes, quartered

1 mango, peeled, stoned and diced

Juice of 1 lime

Handful of coriander, roughly chopped

1. Heat 1 tablespoon of the oil in a large, non-stick pan over a medium heat. Add the onions and cook for 5 minutes until starting to soften. Add the sliced peppers and cook for 5 more minutes, until they have defrosted and started to brown. Remove to a bowl and return the pan to the heat.

2. Heat the remaining oil in the pan. Add the black beans and the liquid from their tins along with the chopped tomatoes. Cook over a high heat until reduced to a thick mixture, around 3 minutes, then stir in the spices and remove from the heat.

3. Mix all the salsa ingredients together in a small bowl.

4. Divide the rice between 4 bowls. Top with the cooked beans, pepper-onion mixture, mashed avocado, lettuce, salsa and drizzle with the hot sauce.

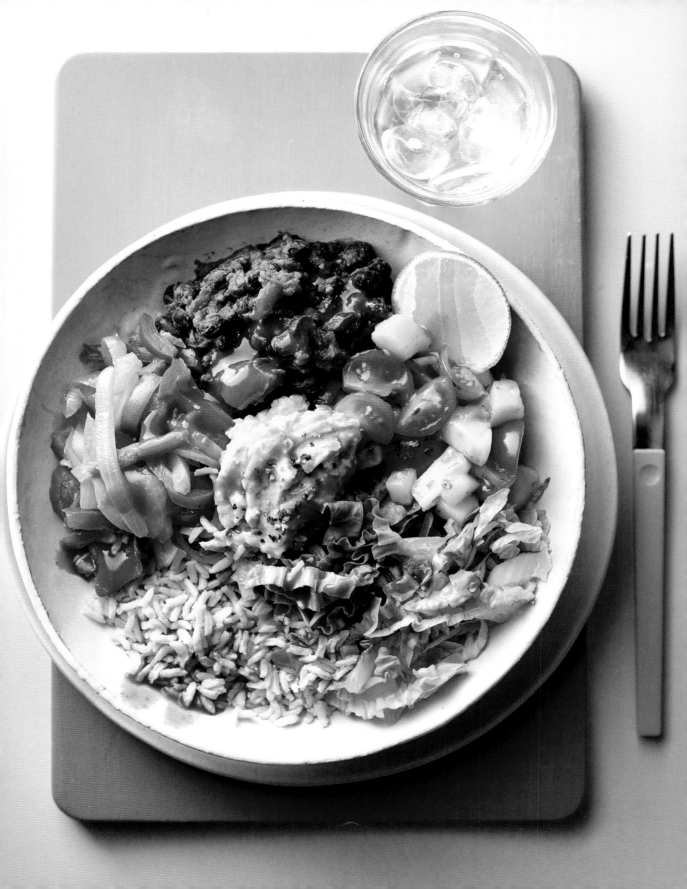

Magic Bean Stew

This super versatile and cheap stew can be changed up to suit your mood and appetite; follow the adaptations for spicy Mexican, Indian and Spanish flavours, or a herby Italian version.

SERVES 12 • 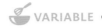 VARIABLE • VARIABLE •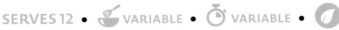

4 tbsp olive oil

4 onions, diced

3 peppers, deseeded and diced, or 350g frozen sliced peppers

6 carrots, diced

6 celery sticks, diced

2 x 400g tins kidney beans

2 x 400g tins black beans

2 x 400g tins cannellini beans

2 x 400g tins chopped tomatoes

1¼ litres water

1 tbsp dried oregano

2 vegetable stock cubes

1. Heat the oil in a large pan over a medium heat. Add the onions, peppers, carrots and celery then cook, stirring occasionally, until softened – around 10 minutes. Add all the beans with their liquid, the tomatoes, water, oregano and the flavourings you are using (see below). Crumble in the stock cubes and stir. Bring to the boil, turn down the heat and simmer for 30 minutes to let the flavours develop.

For Mexican Bean Stew

Add 2 tbsp smoked paprika, 1 tbsp ground cumin, 1 tsp ground cinnamon and 1 tsp chilli flakes. Garnish with chopped fresh coriander.
Eat with: Wholemeal tortillas or brown rice.

For Indian Bean Stew

Leave out the oregano. Add 2 tbsp grated ginger and 6 crushed garlic cloves with the veg. Stir in a 400g tin coconut milk, 2 tbsp garam masala, 2 tsp ground cumin, 2 tsp smoked paprika and 1 tsp chilli powder.
Eat with: Wholemeal flatbreads, natural yoghurt or brown rice.

For Spanish Bean Stew

Stir in 1 tbsp smoked paprika and 160g pitted olives. Before serving, stir in 260g baby spinach and wilt.
Eat with: Crusty ciabatta for dipping.

For Italian Bean Stew

Add 1 tbsp chopped rosemary, 20g chopped basil.
Eat with: Spaghetti, or use as a base for lasagne.

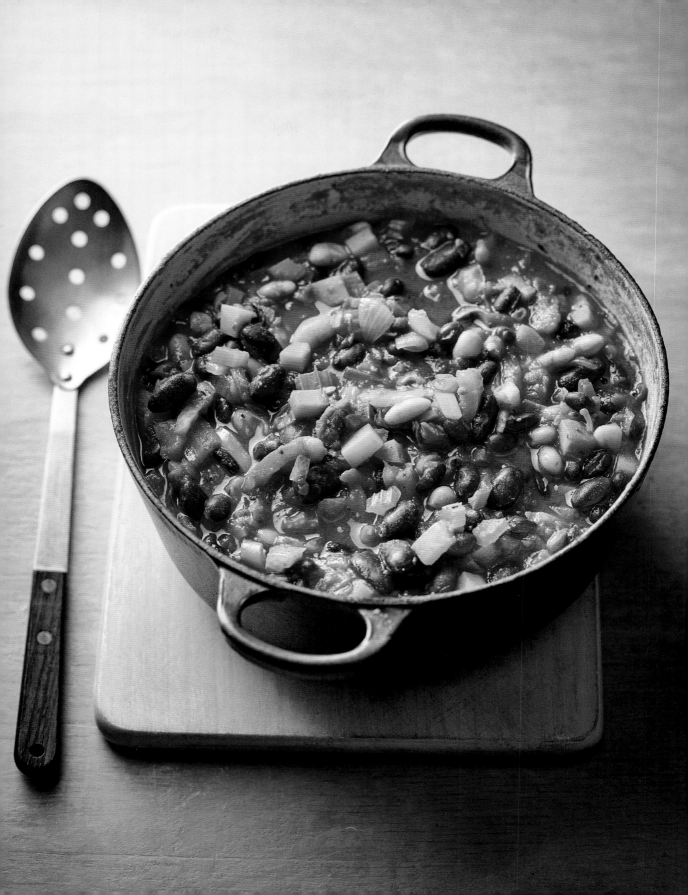

Mushroom 'Kebab' Wraps

This meat-free fakeaway uses thickly sliced mushrooms for their meaty texture and savoury flavour, which is boosted with earthy spices and a healthy, creamy yoghurt dressing.

SERVES 4 • 15 MINS • 25 MINS • V

600g portobello mushrooms, sliced

2 tbsp olive oil

2 garlic cloves, crushed

2 tbsp tomato purée

1 tbsp lemon juice

1 tbsp soy sauce

1½ tsp ground cumin

1 tsp smoked paprika

FOR THE TZATZIKI

150g Greek yoghurt

1 garlic clove, crushed

Handful of fresh mint leaves, finely chopped

Pinch of salt

½ cucumber, finely diced

TO SERVE

4 wholemeal tortillas or wraps, warmed

200g cherry tomatoes, roughly chopped

Handful of parsley, roughly chopped

Mixed salad leaves

1. Preheat the oven to 220°C/200°C fan/425°F/gas mark 7 and line a baking tray with baking paper.

2. Toss the mushrooms with the oil, garlic, tomato purée, lemon juice, soy sauce, cumin and smoked paprika. Spread out on the lined tray and roast for 15–25 minutes, stirring the mushrooms halfway through, until browned.

3. Meanwhile, make the tzatziki by mixing the yoghurt, garlic, mint and salt in a small bowl. Fold in the diced cucumber.

4. Serve the wraps filled with the mushrooms, tzatziki, chopped tomatoes, parsley and salad leaves.

Sesame Tuna Rice Bowls

A complete meal in a bowl! This delicious rice bowl contains proteins, wholegrains, vitamins and omega 3 from the tuna and is really quick to pull together.

SERVES 4 • 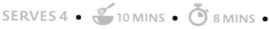 10 MINS • 8 MINS •

4 tbsp sesame seeds

¼ tsp chilli flakes

Pinch of salt

4 tuna steaks

1 tbsp vegetable oil

500g cooked brown rice

2 avocados, pitted and cut into cubes

½ cucumber, thinly sliced

1 medium carrot, cut into matchsticks or coarsely grated

250g frozen peas, defrosted

Handful of coriander, roughly chopped

FOR THE DRESSING

2 tbsp soy sauce

½ tbsp runny honey

½ tbsp apple cider vinegar

1 tsp sesame oil

½ tsp grated fresh ginger

1 spring onion, thinly sliced

1. Combine the sesame seeds, chilli flakes and salt in a shallow bowl. Dip each tuna steak into the sesame seeds, turning to coat both sides.

2. Heat the vegetable oil over a high heat in a non-stick pan. Once hot, add 2 of the tuna steaks and cook for 1½–2 minutes per side, until cooked on the outside but still pink in the centre. Remove to a board and cut into 2cm cubes. Repeat with the remaining tuna steaks.

3. Combine the dressing ingredients in a jar and shake to combine.

4. Divide the rice between 4 bowls and top with the cubed tuna, avocado, cucumber, carrot, peas and coriander. Drizzle over the dressing and serve.

Dal with Spinach Flatbreads

Lentils are packed with protein and prebiotic fibre and are so easy to cook. The spinach flatbreads are perfect for scooping up the dal and a clever way to get more veg into your diet.

SERVES 4 • 25 MINS • 50 MINS • V

1½ tbsp coconut oil or vegetable oil

2 banana shallots, thinly sliced

2 garlic cloves, crushed

1 tbsp grated fresh ginger

2 tsp cumin seeds

200g red lentils

1 litre water

1 x 400g tin chopped tomatoes

1 tsp garam masala

Pinch of salt

FOR THE FLATBREADS

250g baby spinach

150g natural yoghurt

250g self-raising flour, plus extra for dusting

Pinch of salt

1 tbsp vegetable oil or melted coconut oil

TIP
If you don't have self-raising flour, use an equal weight of plain flour mixed with 2 tsp baking powder.

1. Heat 1 tablespoon of the oil in a large pan over a medium-low heat and cook the shallots until golden, 7–10 minutes. Remove from the pan and set aside.

2. Add the remaining oil to the pan with the garlic, ginger and cumin seeds. Cook for 1–2 minutes until fragrant then add the lentils, water and tomatoes. Bring to a boil then lower to a simmer. Cook for 20–30 minutes, until the lentils are tender, then stir in the garam masala and remove from the heat. Taste and season with salt, then mix in the cooked shallots.

3. For the flatbreads, place the spinach in a colander set over the sink. Boil the kettle and pour the boiling water over the spinach to wilt it. Rinse under cold running water to cool, then squeeze the spinach with your hands to remove as much water as possible.

4. Weigh 100g of the squeezed spinach (any excess spinach can be stirred into the dal) and blitz with the yoghurt. Stir in the flour and salt to a slightly sticky dough. Cover and set aside for 30 minutes.

5. Divide the dough into 8 and roll each piece out to 3mm thick on a flour-dusted surface. Dust off excess flour then brush the flatbreads with oil. Cook, oiled side down, in a hot frying or griddle pan over a high heat until golden underneath. Brush the other side of the flatbread with oil, flip, then cook until golden. Keep warm while you cook the remaining flatbreads.

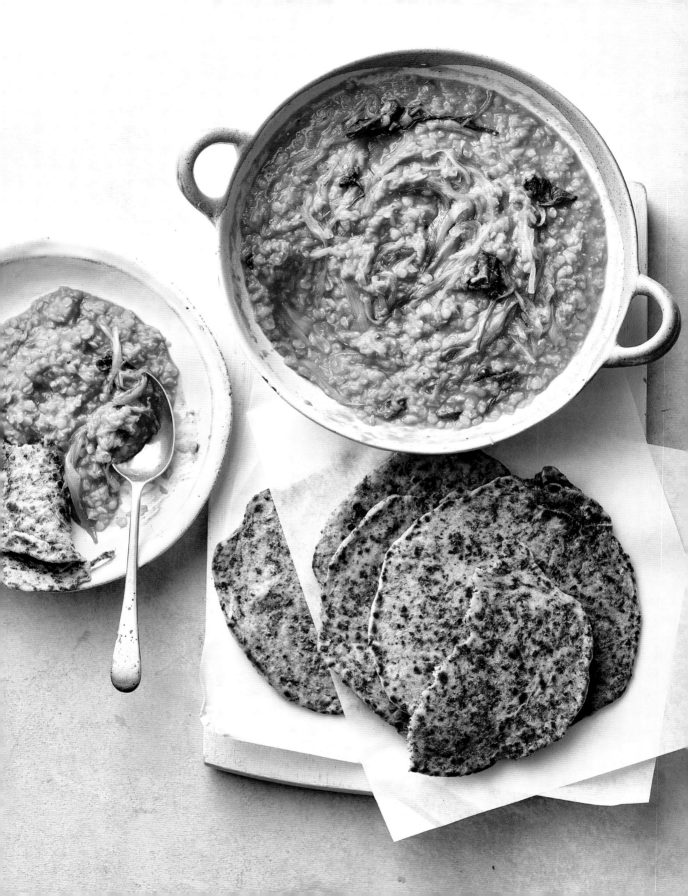

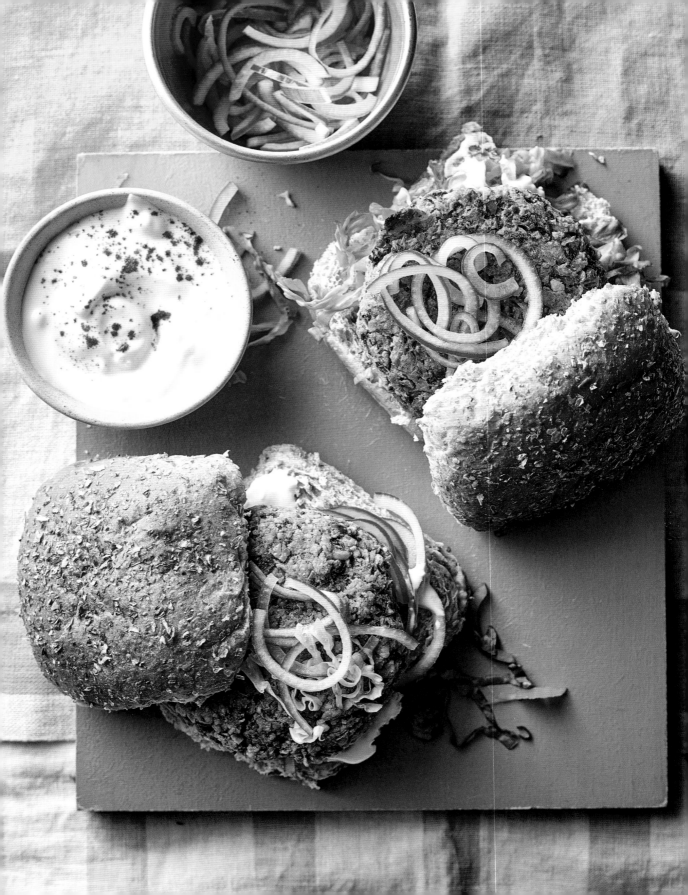

Falafel Burgers

These meat-free burgers make a delicious, low-fat and nutritious alternative to traditional meat burgers, and are full of spicy flavours, topped with a creamy yoghurt sauce.

MAKES 8 BURGERS • 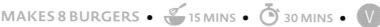 15 MINS • 30 MINS • V

2 tbsp extra virgin olive oil
2 small red onions
Juice of ½ lemon
60g coriander leaves
2 tsp ground cumin
2 tsp garlic granules
1 tsp ground coriander
1 egg
2 x 400g tins chickpeas, drained
and rinsed
100g frozen peas, defrosted
50g golden breadcrumbs
3 tbsp plain white flour
Pinch of salt

FOR THE YOGHURT SAUCE
4 tbsp natural yoghurt
1 garlic clove, crushed
Juice of ½ lemon

TO SERVE
8 wholemeal buns, split and toasted
1 head gem lettuce, finely shredded

1. Preheat the oven to 200°C/180°C fan/400°F/gas mark 6, line a baking tray with baking paper and brush with 1 tablespoon of the olive oil.

2. Thinly slice one of the onions and place into a bowl. Squeeze over the lemon juice and set aside for a few minutes to turn pink.

3. Meanwhile, roughly chop the other onion and add to a food processor along with the leaves of the fresh coriander. Finely chop the coriander stalks and add them in too, along with the cumin, garlic granules, ground coriander and egg. Blitz to a coarse paste. Add the chickpeas and peas and pulse to a chunky mixture.

4. Scrape the mixture into a bowl and mix in the breadcrumbs, flour and salt. Divide the mixture into 8 balls and flatten onto the baking tray. Bake for 20–30 minutes, flipping the patties halfway through, until slightly browned.

5. Mix together the yoghurt sauce ingredients in a small bowl.

6. Spread some yoghurt sauce on the bottom half of each split bun, top with the pattie, the shredded lettuce and a few of the reserved onion slices. Pop on the bun lid and serve straight away.

Veggie Korma

This curry is so good you'll wonder why you ever ordered a takeaway. Filled with delicous veg and cooked in a low-fat, lightly spiced coconut-milk sauce, this is a delicious, cheap supper.

SERVES 4 • 15 MINS • 40 MINS •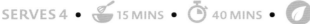

1 head cauliflower, separated into florets

2 tbsp melted coconut oil or vegetable oil

2 onions, diced

1 tbsp grated fresh ginger

4 garlic cloves, crushed

4 green cardamom pods, bashed

½ tsp ground coriander

½ tsp ground cinnamon

½ tsp ground turmeric

2 tomatoes, diced

1 x 400g tin light coconut milk

500ml water

2 tsp garam masala

200g green beans, trimmed

100g frozen peas

500g cooked brown basmati rice

Sprigs of fresh coriander, for garnish

FOR THE QUICK MANGO PICKLE

1 mango, peeled, stoned and diced

Juice of 1 lime

¼ tsp curry powder

Pinch of salt

1. Preheat the oven to 200°C/180°C fan/400°F/gas mark 6.

2. For the mango pickle, combine the diced mango, lime juice, curry powder and salt in a small bowl. Stir together then set aside while you make the curry.

3. Toss the cauliflower florets with 1 tablespoon of the oil on a large baking tray. Place into the oven to roast for 25–35 minutes, until golden.

4. Meanwhile, heat the remaining 1 tablespoon of oil in a medium pan over a medium-low heat. Add the onions and cook until starting to turn golden, about 7–10 minutes. Stir in the ginger, garlic and cardamom pods for 1–2 minutes until fragrant. Stir in the ground coriander, cinnamon and turmeric, the tomatoes, coconut milk and water. Bring to a simmer then allow to cook over a low heat for 10 minutes so the flavours can infuse and the tomatoes have softened.

5. Remove from the heat and stir in the garam masala, then blitz the mixture until smooth. Return to the heat and add the green beans to the pan, letting them cook for 4–5 minutes until tender. Finally, stir in the peas and roasted cauliflower.

6. Serve with the rice and the mango pickle on the side, garnished with a few sprigs of coriander.

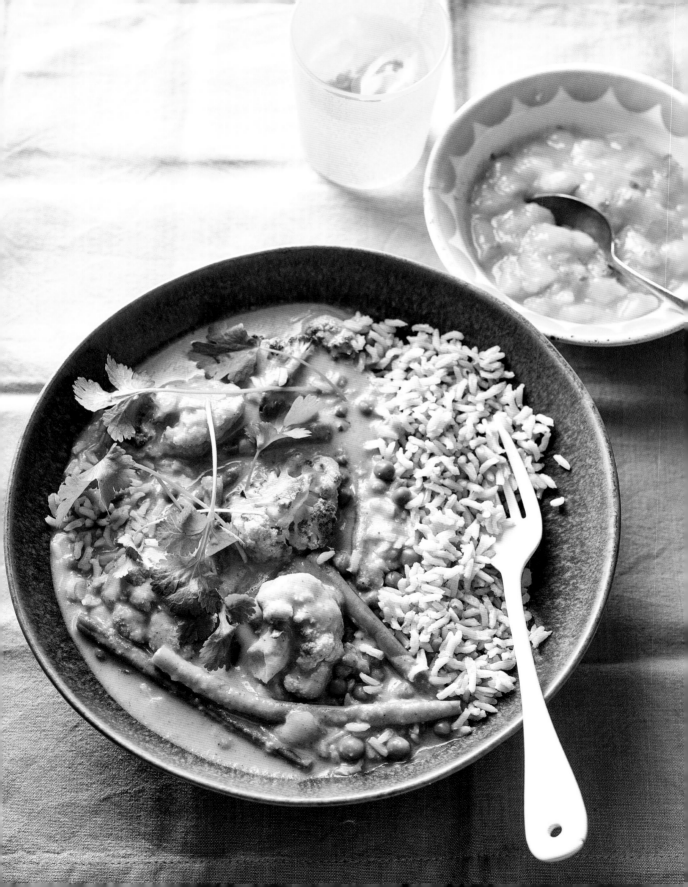

Green Barley Risotto

Barley is the perfect rice alternative here. It has more fibre and protein than rice, slowly releasing energy, while kale is a vitamin and mineral powerhouse.

SERVES 4 • 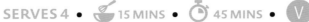 15 MINS • 45 MINS • V

2 tbsp olive oil

2 onions, finely diced

2 carrots, finely diced

3 celery sticks, finely diced

300g pearl barley

4 sprigs of thyme

1 bay leaf

1¼ litres vegetable stock

200g frozen peas

100g baby spinach

30g Parmesan cheese, finely grated

40g walnuts, roughly chopped

FOR THE KALE PESTO

40g chopped curly kale

30g basil leaves

75ml extra virgin olive oil

Zest and juice of 1 lemon

1 garlic clove, crushed

2 tbsp sunflower seeds

Pinch of salt

1. Heat the oil in a medium pan over a medium heat. Add the onions, carrots and celery, then cook until softened, around 10 minutes. Add the pearl barley and cook for 2 minutes more, to toast. Add the thyme, bay leaf and 500ml of the stock. Bring to the boil then turn down to simmer and cook, stirring occasionally, until the liquid is mostly absorbed, about 20 minutes. Add the remaining stock, bring back to the boil and turn down to simmer. Allow to cook, stirring occasionally, until the barley is tender – 10–15 minutes. If it's looking too dry, top up with more water.

2. Remove the bay leaf and thyme sprigs, stir in the peas and spinach until warmed through and wilted then remove from the heat.

3. For the kale pesto, blitz the kale, basil, oil, lemon zest and juice, garlic, sunflower seeds and salt in a food processor until finely chopped. Thin with water until you get a drizzleable consistency.

4. Serve the barley risotto topped with a spoonful of pesto, the grated Parmesan and chopped walnuts.

Aubergine Meatballs

Aubergine makes a fantastic plant-based mince alternative, and this is a really interesting dish to try. These 'meatballs' can be prepped ahead and frozen, ready to cook as needed.

SERVES 4 • 20 MINS • 45 MINS •

2 aubergines (around 500g), cut into 3cm chunks

4 tbsp extra virgin olive oil

1 red onion, roughly chopped

1 x 400g tin black beans, drained and rinsed

80g porridge oats

60g dry breadcrumbs

1 tsp garlic granules

1 tsp dried oregano

1 egg

2 x 400g tins chopped tomatoes

1 tbsp balsamic vinegar

Handful of fresh basil, roughly chopped

300g wholemeal spaghetti

30g Parmesan cheese, finely grated, to serve

Salt

1. Preheat the oven to 200°C/180°C fan/400°F/gas mark 6.

2. Toss the aubergine chunks with 1 tablespoon of the oil and a pinch of salt on a large baking tray. Bake for 25–30 minutes until soft and turning golden.

3. Add the onion to a food processor and blitz until quite finely chopped. Add the cooked aubergine chunks and blend until pureed. Add the black beans and pulse until roughly chopped with some whole beans remaining. Scrape into a bowl and stir in the oats, breadcrumbs, garlic granules and oregano. Taste and season with salt then stir in the egg.

4. Roll heaped tablespoons of the mixture into balls. Place on the same tray you were using before, spacing them a few centimetres apart. Drizzle with 2 tablespoons of the oil and bake for 15 minutes.

5. Meanwhile, heat the remaining oil in a medium pan over a medium heat. Add the tomatoes, balsamic vinegar, basil and a pinch of salt. Bring to a boil, turn the heat down to low and leave to cook for 15–20 minutes, stirring occasionally, until slightly thickened.

6. Bring a large pan of water to the boil and cook the spaghetti according to the instructions on the packet. Drain and return to the pan. Toss some of the tomato sauce through the pasta then divide between 4 bowls. Mix the meatballs into the remaining sauce then divide between the bowls and sprinkle with cheese.

Cauliflower Mac & Cheese

Mac & cheese is an easy family favourite, but using cauliflower too adds texture and fibre. Using mature rather than mild cheese has the same flavour but uses less, keeping fat levels low.

SERVES 4 • 15 MINS • 45 MINS •

700g (1 large) cauliflower, cut into florets

3 tbsp extra virgin olive oil

300g wholemeal penne pasta

45g plain white flour

350ml milk

200ml water

1 tsp Worcestershire sauce or Marmite

¼ tsp smoked paprika

¼ tsp garlic granules

2 tsp lemon juice

120g mature Cheddar cheese, grated

3 tbsp breadcrumbs

Salt and freshly ground black pepper

1. Preheat the oven to 200°C/180°C fan/400°F/gas mark 6.

2. Toss the cauliflower florets with 1 tablespoon of olive oil in a 23 x 33cm roasting dish then roast for 30 minutes until soft and starting to brown.

3. Bring a large pan of salted water to the boil and cook the pasta according to the instructions on the packet. Drain. Turn the oven up to 240°C/220°C fan/475°F/gas mark 9.

4. Meanwhile, heat the remaining olive oil in a medium pan over a high heat. Add the flour and stir for 2 minutes. Gradually pour in the milk, whisking well. Stir in the water, Worcestershire sauce or Marmite, smoked paprika, garlic granules, lemon juice and cheese and cook until the cheese has melted. Taste and season as needed. Remove from the heat.

5. Add half of the roasted cauliflower to the cheese sauce, tip into a blender and blend until smooth.

6. Tip the pasta into the roasting dish containing the whole cauliflower florets. Pour the sauce over and stir to coat. Sprinkle with the breadcrumbs and bake for 7–10 minutes, until the sauce starts to bubble.

7. Heat the grill and cook for 2–4 minutes until the breadcrumbs have browned. Serve hot.

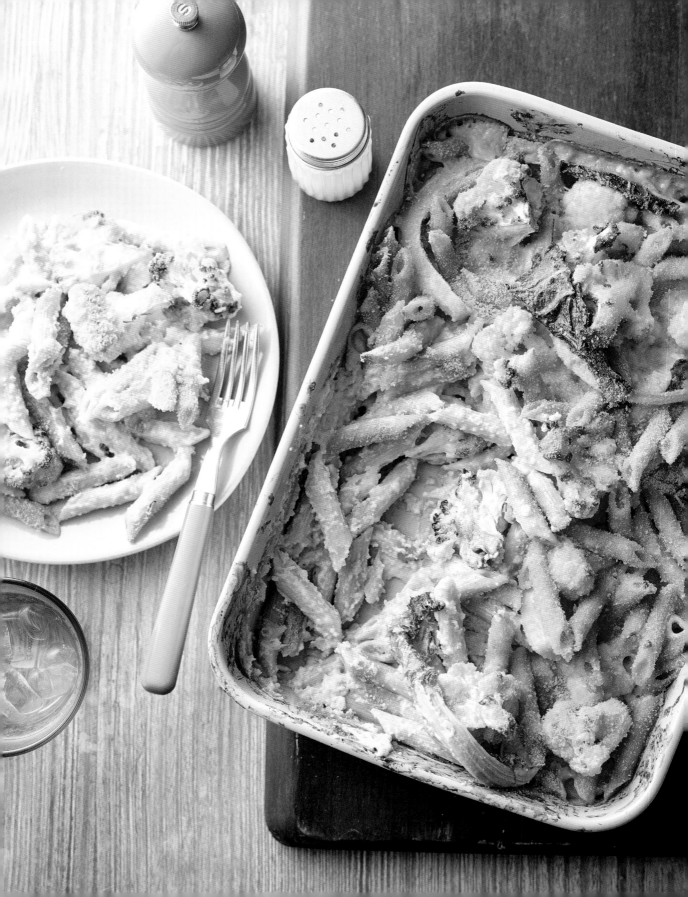

Sardine, Tomato & Chilli Pasta

Perfect for a busy weeknight supper, this pasta sauce uses storecupboard standbys of tinned sardines, beans and cherry tomatoes, for a filling and nutritious bowl.

SERVES 4 • 10 MINS • 25 MINS •

4 garlic cloves, roughly chopped

½ tsp chilli flakes

2 x 90g tin sardines packed in olive oil, reserve the oil

1 x 400g tin cannellini beans

2 x 400g tin cherry tomatoes

50g tomato purée

2 tsp capers, roughly chopped

½ tsp granulated sugar

300g wholemeal spaghetti

Handful of fresh parsley, roughly chopped

1. In a large, non-stick frying pan set over a medium heat, sauté the garlic and chilli flakes in 1 tablespoon of the oil from the sardine tins. After 1 minute, add the sardines, then once the garlic is starting to turn golden and the sardines are softening, add the beans and their liquid from the tin to the pan. Cook until the liquid has reduced down a bit then add tomatoes, tomato purée, capers and sugar. Stir together, then turn the heat down to low. Cook for 15–20 minutes, stirring occasionally, until the sauce is thick and jammy.

2. Meanwhile, bring a large pan of salted water to the boil. Add the pasta and cook according to the packet instructions. Use tongs to transfer the cooked pasta directly from the pot into the frying pan. Add a splash of the pasta cooking water and toss together with the tongs to coat the pasta with the sauce.

3. Divide between 4 bowls and serve sprinkled with some parsley.

TIP

If you don't like sardines, try using an equal weight of tuna packed in olive oil instead.

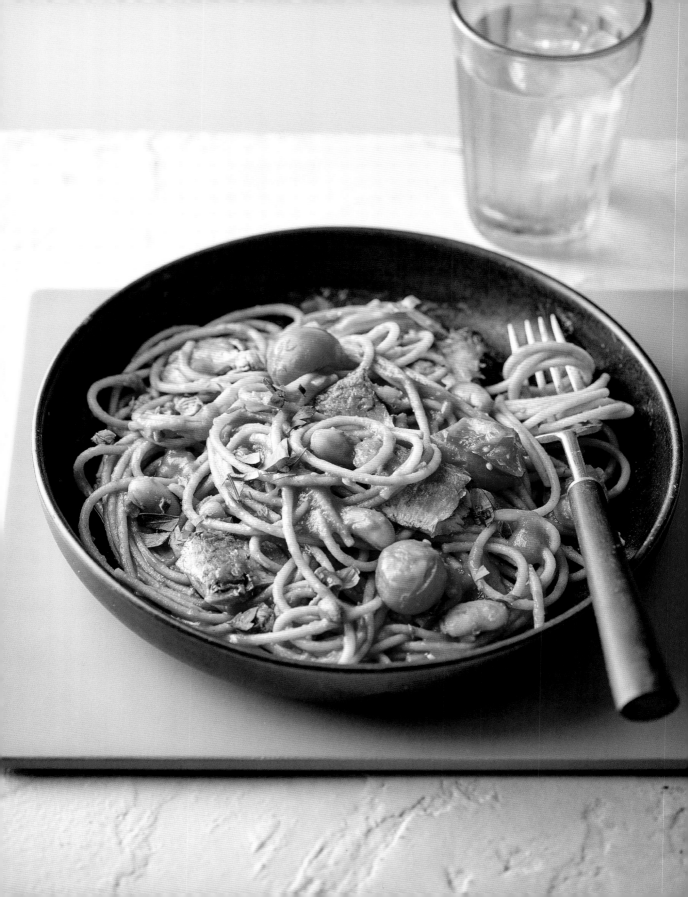

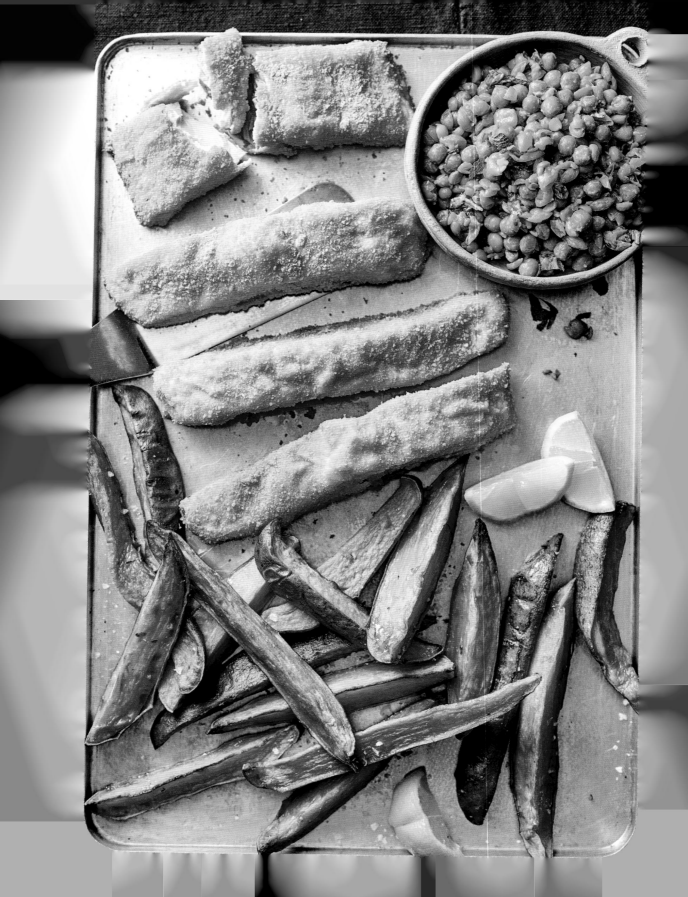

Baked Salmon with Sweet Potato Wedges & Mushy Peas

An easy twist on traditional fish fingers, these homemade versions are baked rather than fried, which keeps the fat level low, and are served with vitamin- and mineral-rich sweet potatoes.

SERVES 4 • 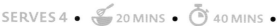 20 MINS • 40 MINS •

FOR THE SWEET POTATO WEDGES
3 sweet potatoes (600g), peeled and cut into wedges

1 tbsp olive oil

Salt

FOR THE FISH
50g plain white flour

1 egg, beaten

80g golden breadcrumbs

4 x 150g salmon fillets (or each of a similar weight)

1 tbsp olive oil

1 lemon, thickly sliced

FOR THE MUSHY PEAS
300g frozen peas

1 tbsp finely chopped fresh mint leaves

1 tbsp butter

1 tsp lemon juice

1. Preheat the oven to 200°C/180°C fan/400°F/gas mark 6.

2. Toss the sweet potato wedges with the oil and salt on a large baking tray. Roast for 30–40 minutes, flipping them over halfway through, until soft and golden.

3. Meanwhile, place the flour, egg and breadcrumbs into three separate shallow dishes. To the beaten egg, add 2 tablespoons of water.

4. Dip each salmon fillet into the flour to coat, shaking off any excess, then into the egg and then the breadcrumbs, to evenly coat.

5. Place the breadcrumbed salmon onto a baking tray. Drizzle with the oil and bake for 12–15 minutes, until the fish flakes apart easily and is cooked through.

6. Place the peas in a bowl and cover with boiling water. Set aside for 5 minutes, drain and return to the bowl, then add the mint and butter. Mash briefly with a potato masher until you get a chunky paste. Stir in the lemon juice and a pinch of salt.

7. Serve the salmon with the wedges and peas on the side. Garnish with a couple of lemon slices.

Soy & Ginger Steamed Haddock Parcels

Steaming is a healthy way to cook, conserving more nutrients then other cooking techniques. Serving the fish and cabbage with brown rice makes this a nutritionally complete meal.

SERVES 4 • 10 MINS • 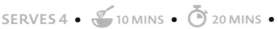 20 MINS •

1 small or ½ large head Savoy cabbage, cut into 12 wedges

1 lime, zested then thinly sliced

4 x 130g haddock fillets

1 red chilli, deseeded and finely diced

2 tsp grated fresh ginger

3 spring onions, finely sliced

4 tsp extra virgin olive oil

2 tbsp soy sauce

500g brown basmati rice

1. Preheat the oven to 200°C/180°C fan/400°F/gas mark 6. Take 2 large pieces of tin foil and lay equal-sized pieces of baking paper on top of them.

2. Divide the cabbage wedges between the two pieces of baking paper. Top with the slices of lime followed by the haddock fillets. Sprinkle with the lime zest, diced chilli, grated ginger and sliced spring onions. Drizzle 1 teaspoon of olive oil over each piece of fish then drizzle the soy sauce over everything.

3. Fold the baking paper and foil over the fish, ensuring you fold the edges together to seal tightly. Place both parcels onto a large baking tray and bake for 15–20 minutes, depending on the thickness of the haddock, until the fish flakes apart easily.

4. Meanwhile, cook the rice in a pan of boiling water, following the instructions on the packet.

5. Serve the fish and cabbage alongside the rice, pouring any juice from the parcels on top.

TIPS

Swap the haddock for another white fish or salmon fillets.

Change the cabbage to pak choi, asparagus, Tenderstem broccoli or green beans.

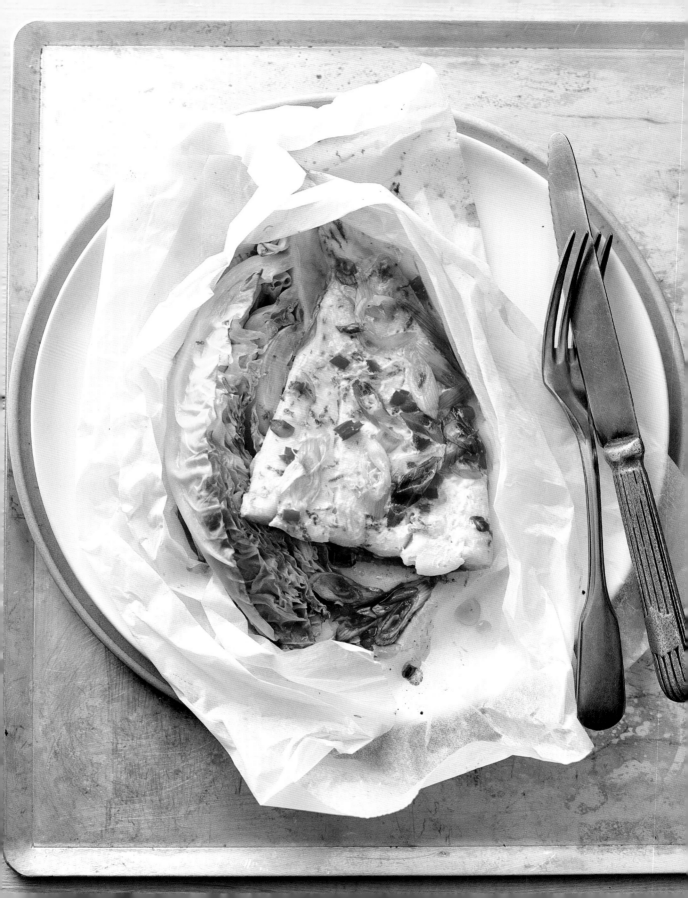

Teriyaki Salmon

A fresh and tasty way to serve salmon; the teriyaki sauce with added dates makes a fibre-filled sauce, and blitzing broccoli into the rice is a clever way to increase the veg count.

SERVES 4 • 🥄 15 MINS • ⏱ 25 MINS •

4 x 120g salmon fillets, skin on
1 head broccoli
1 tbsp vegetable oil
200g green beans, trimmed
Pinch of salt
500g cooked brown basmati rice
1 tbsp sesame seeds, to garnish

FOR THE DATE TERIYAKI SAUCE

50g pitted dates, soaked in boiling
    water for 10 minutes
1 tsp garlic granules
2 tsp grated fresh ginger
3 tbsp orange juice
4 tbsp soy sauce
1 tsp sesame oil
1 tbsp cornflour
3 tbsp water
1 tsp runny honey
2 tsp apple cider vinegar

TIP
Any leftover sauce can be kept in an airtight container in the fridge for up to 3 days or in the freezer for up to 3 months.

1. Preheat the oven to 220°C/200°C fan/425°F/gas mark 7 and line a baking tray with baking paper.

2. Drain the soaked dates then blitz with the remaining teriyaki sauce ingredients to get a smooth paste. Transfer to a small pan and cook over a low heat, stirring constantly, until thickened and glossy. Remove from the heat and set aside.

3. Place the salmon skin-side down onto the lined baking tray and place in the oven. Bake for 10 minutes then spoon 1 tablespoon of the teriyaki sauce over each fillet. Return to the oven for 2–5 minutes, until the salmon is cooked through.

4. Separate the broccoli into florets and place in a food processor. Blitz to a rice-like texture, set aside. If you don't have a food processor, you can finely shred the broccoli with a knife, working from the flowery top down towards the stem.

5. Heat half the oil in a large, non-stick frying pan over a high heat. Once hot, add the green beans and the salt then sauté until charred and slightly soft, around 5 minutes. Remove the beans from the pan.

6. Add the remaining oil to the pan and stir in the broccoli. Cook until softened and vibrant green, around 5 minutes, then stir in the cooked rice and remove from the heat.

7. Serve the broccoli rice with the salmon and green beans, sprinkled with sesame seeds. The extra teriyaki sauce can be served on the side, as needed.

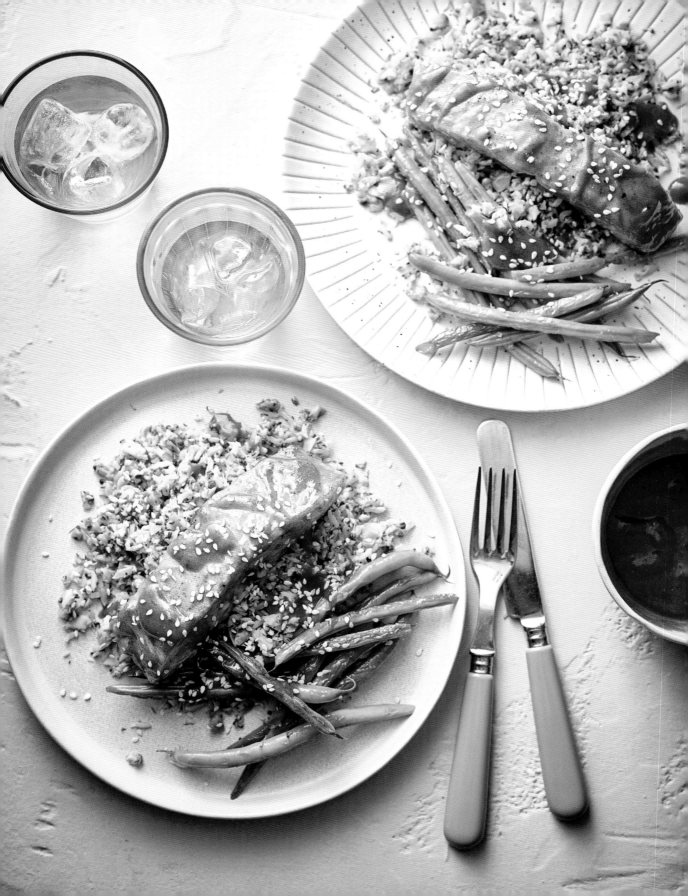

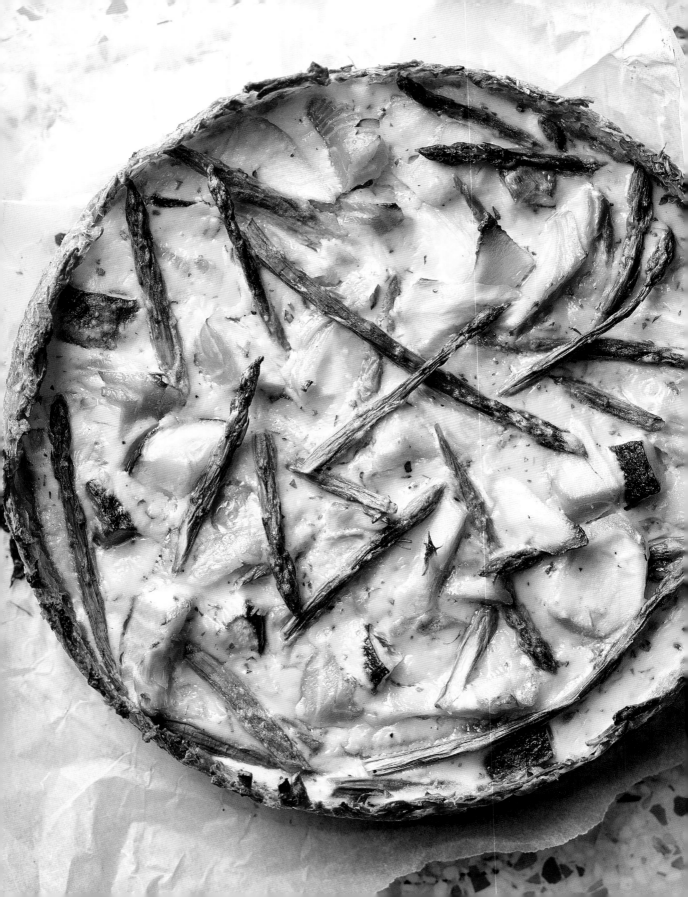

Salmon, Asparagus & Courgette Quiche

Using potatoes in the pastry crust for this quiche instead of butter provides a healthy source of starchy carbohydrates but is lower in fat. The asparagus gives a good vitamin C boost.

SERVES 4–6 • 25 MINS • 1 HR 10 MINS • ❄

FOR THE POTATO CRUST

650g potatoes, coarsely grated

1 tbsp extra virgin olive oil

2 tbsp wholemeal plain flour

FOR THE FILLING

2 medium courgettes, cut into 3-cm chunks

1 tbsp extra virgin olive oil

250g asparagus, woody ends removed then cut in half crosswise

6 large eggs

250g ricotta cheese

4 sprigs of thyme, leaves picked

240g hot-smoked salmon or trout fillets

Salt and freshly ground black pepper

TIP

If you can't find hot-smoked salmon or trout, use salmon. Wrap 2 x 120g salmon fillets in foil and bake in the oven at 200°C/180°C fan/400°F/gas mark 6 for 15 minutes, until the fish flakes. Peel and discard the skin.

1. Preheat the oven to 200°C/180°C fan/400°F/gas mark 6. Set a 23cm springform cake tin onto a baking tray. Line the base of the tin with baking paper.

2. Spread the grated potatoes out over a cutting board and sprinkle with salt, set aside for 5 minutes. Transfer the grated potatoes to a clean tea towel, twist the edges of the towel together at the top and squeeze over the sink to remove as much liquid as possible. Tip into a bowl with 1 tablespoon of the olive oil and the flour. Mix together, then sprinkle into the tin, pressing the potato mixture evenly over the base and 4cm up the sides. Try not to leave any gaps. Bake for 30–35 minutes until the potato is starting to turn golden.

3. Reduce the oven temperature to 180°C/160°C fan/350°F/gas mark 4.

4. Meanwhile, sauté the courgettes with the olive oil in a medium frying pan over medium-low heat, stirring occasionally, until browned – around 15 minutes. In the final 2 minutes of the courgettes cooking, add the asparagus to the frying pan so it can soften slightly.

5. In a medium bowl, whisk the eggs, ricotta and thyme leaves with a pinch each of salt and pepper.

6. Flake the fish and scatter over the potato crust. Top with the cooked courgettes and pour over the beaten egg mixture. Top with the asparagus then bake for 25–35 minutes, until the egg has set.

Prawn & Brown Rice Stir-fry

When you want dinner on the table fast, this is a great choice. Fibre-filled brown rice takes longer to cook than noodles, but is more nutritious, boosted by a rainbow of coloured veg.

SERVES 4 • 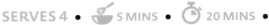 5 MINS • 20 MINS •

200g brown rice
1 tbsp vegetable oil
1 tbsp sesame oil
2 peppers, deseeded and sliced
200g baby corn, roughly chopped
200g mangetout
200g green beans, trimmed
100g frozen peas
300g cooked, peeled king prawns
1 tbsp grated fresh ginger
3 garlic cloves, crushed
3 tbsp soy sauce
1 tbsp runny honey
4 spring onions, thinly sliced

1. Place the brown rice into a medium pan and cover well with boiling water. Place over a high heat and bring to the boil, turn down to simmer and cook for 20 minutes until tender. Drain the rice and return to the pan, and cover with a lid. Leave to stand for 5 minutes so it can steam.

2. Meanwhile, heat the vegetable and sesame oils in a large, non-stick frying pan or wok over a high heat. Once hot, add the peppers, corn, mangetout and green beans. Stir-fry until the vegetables have softened and are starting to char in places – around 5 minutes. Add the peas and prawns then cook for 1–2 minutes until warmed through.

3. Mix the ginger, garlic, soy and honey in a small bowl. Pour into the pan along with the rice and stir everything to coat. Divide between 4 bowls and top with the sliced spring onions.

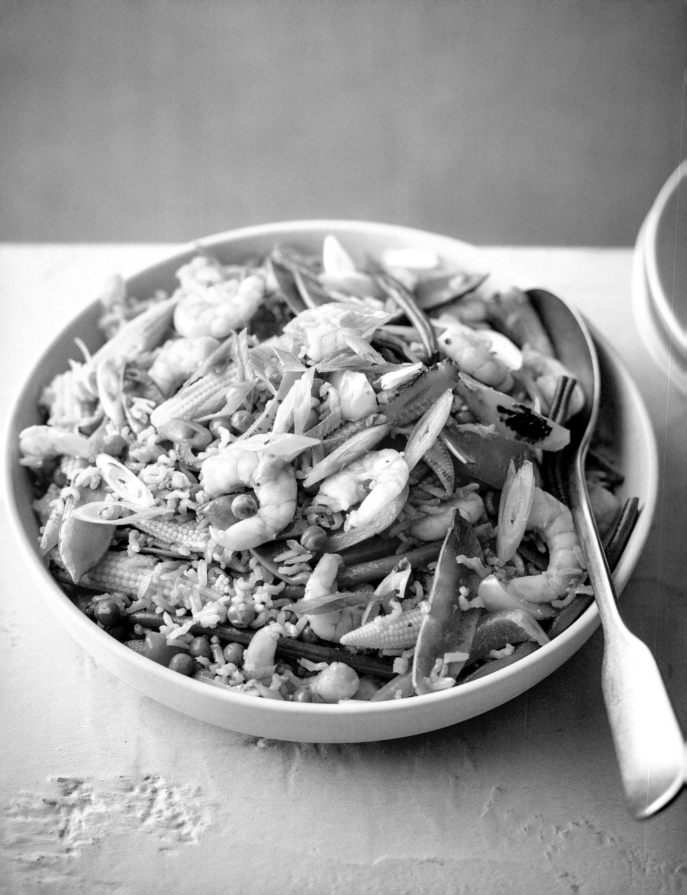

Sweet & Sour Chicken

Another brilliant fakeaway that you can cook quicker than it takes to order a delivery – and it's much healthier too! Make it yourself and you can add extra veg and keep salt and fat levels low.

SERVES 4 • 20 MINS • 20 MINS •

2 tbsp vegetable oil

4 chicken breasts, cut into bite-sized chunks

3 peppers, deseeded and diced

1 small head broccoli, cut into bite-sized florets

150g frozen peas

500g cooked brown basmati rice

2 spring onions, thinly sliced

FOR THE SWEET AND SOUR SAUCE

150g frozen pineapple chunks

2 tbsp soy sauce

2 tbsp water

1 tbsp runny honey

1 tbsp ketchup

1 tbsp apple cider vinegar

3 garlic cloves, crushed

1 tbsp grated fresh ginger

1 tbsp cornflour

1. Combine the sauce ingredients, except the cornflour, in a small pan. Cover with a lid and place over a medium heat. Leave to cook for 5 minutes to soften the pineapple, then blitz until mostly smooth using a hand blender in the pan (alternatively, use a free-standing blender or food processor then return it to the pan).

2. Mix 2 tablespoons of the sauce with the cornflour in a small bowl then pour this back into the sauce, stir to mix, then return to the heat until the sauce starts to bubble and has thickened slightly. Remove from the heat and set aside.

3. Heat 1 tablespoon of the oil in a large, non-stick frying pan over a medium heat. Add the chicken chunks and cook until golden all over – around 5–6 minutes – then remove to a plate. Add the remaining oil, the diced peppers and broccoli and cook over a medium-high heat until softened slightly, around 5 minutes. Stir in the peas to defrost, then remove from the heat.

4. Add the chicken and the sauce to the frying pan and stir everything together to coat.

5. Serve the chicken with the rice, garnished with the spring onions.

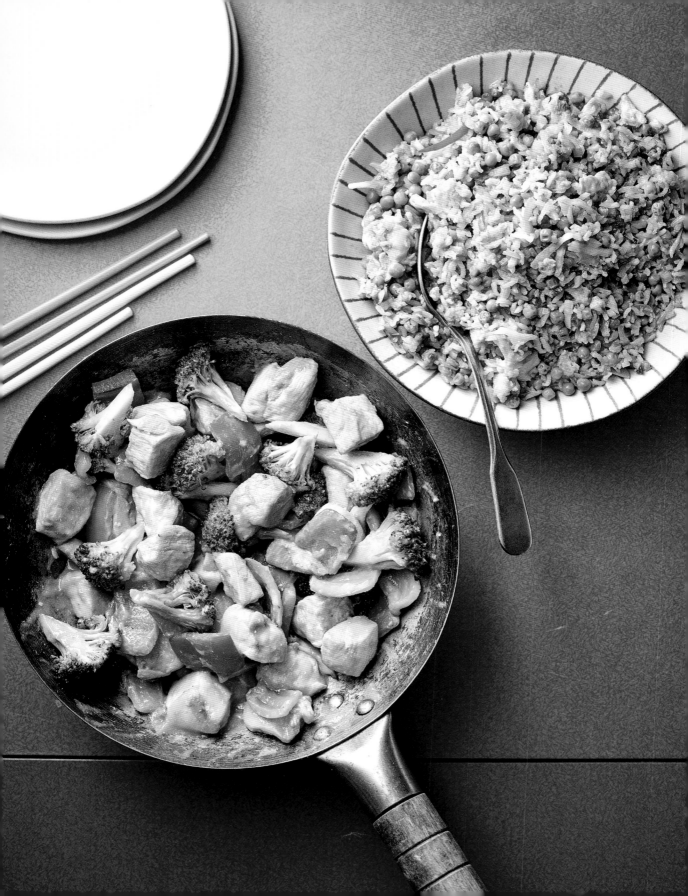

Egg-fried Rice

Cauliflower is a brilliantly versatile ingredient, and here it is blitzed into grains to fill out the rice. You can also add another vegetable into this healthier version of a Chinese takeaway favourite.

SERVES 4 • 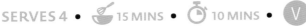 15 MINS • 🕙 10 MINS • Ⓥ

½ head (350g) cauliflower, separated into florets

1 tbsp vegetable oil

1 tsp sesame oil

4 garlic cloves, crushed

1 tbsp grated fresh ginger

1 red chilli, deseeded and finely diced

1 carrot, coarsely grated

½ small or ¼ large head cabbage, finely shredded

2 tbsp soy sauce

1 tbsp oyster sauce (optional)

500g cooked brown rice

150g frozen peas

4 eggs, lightly beaten

3 spring onions, finely sliced

1. Blitz the cauliflower in a food processor until it resembles rice. If you don't have a food processor you can grate the cauliflower on the coarse side of a box grated instead. Set aside.

2. Heat the oils in a large, non-stick frying pan over a high heat. Add the garlic, ginger and chilli then cook for 1 minute to soften. Add the cauliflower and sauté until it has released most of its liquid – around 5 minutes. Stir in the carrot, cabbage, soy sauce and oyster sauce (if using). Stir for 2–3 minutes more, until the cabbage has softened, then mix in the rice and peas.

3. Push the mixture to the sides of the pan, making a hole in the centre, and add the beaten eggs. Stir through the rice and cook until the eggs have set. Serve garnished with the spring onions.

TIP
To make this more filling, add a couple of cooked, shredded chicken breasts or some stir-fried cubes of firm tofu.

Chicken & Courgette Katsu Curry

A warming and satisfying homemade katsu curry with added vegetables. You can double up the breaded chicken and the curry sauce and freeze them separately to get ahead another day.

SERVES 4 • 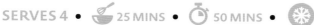 25 MINS • 50 MINS •

3 tbsp olive oil

2 onions, diced

2 carrots, diced

3 garlic cloves, crushed

1 tbsp grated fresh ginger

100g golden breadcrumbs

75g plain white flour

1 egg, beaten

2 courgettes, sliced into 2cm thick coins

3 chicken breasts, cut into 5cm pieces

500g cooked brown basmati rice, to serve

FOR THE CURRY SAUCE

2 tbsp olive oil

40g plain white flour

1 tbsp garam masala

1 tbsp curry powder

600ml low-salt chicken stock or veg stock

1 tbsp soy sauce

2 tsp runny honey

1 tsp apple cider vinegar

1. Preheat the oven to 200°C/180°C fan/400°F/gas mark 6 and line two large baking trays with baking paper then grease each with ½ tablespoon of the oil.

2. Make the sauce. Heat the oil with the flour in a medium pan over a low heat. Cook, stirring, for 10 minutes. Add the garam masala and curry powder then whisk in the stock until smooth. Stir in the soy sauce, honey and vinegar and cook until thickened. Remove from the heat.

3. In a small frying pan, heat 1 tablespoon oil over a medium heat and cook the onions and carrots until the onions are starting to soften and turn golden, 5–7 minutes. Add the garlic and ginger, stir for 1 minute, then pour in the sauce from the pan. Cook over a low heat for 3–5 minutes, stirring occasionally, to soften the vegetables further, then remove from the heat.

4. Place the breadcrumbs, flour and egg into separate, shallow dishes. Mix 2 tablespoons of water into the eggs. Dip the courgette into the flour to coat, shaking off excess, followed by the egg and breadcrumbs. Repeat with the chicken pieces.

5. Lay the courgette on one tray, the chicken on the other. Drizzle with the remaining oil and bake for 25–35 minutes, until golden and crisp, flipping over halfway through the cooking time. Serve the chicken and courgette pieces with the curry sauce and rice.

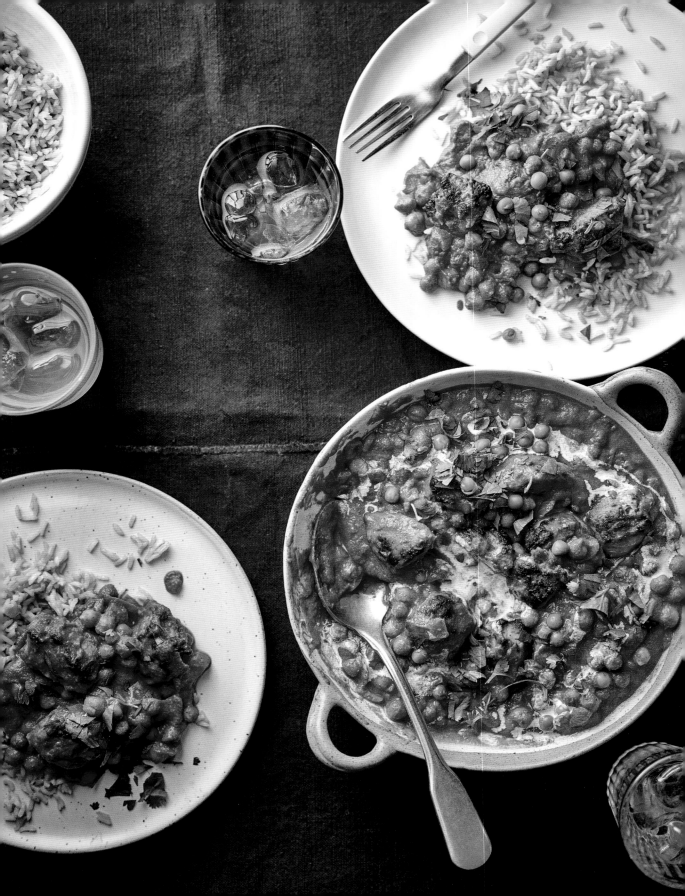

Chicken Tikka Masala

Enjoy the spicy kick of this favourite curry in this lighter version that's lower in fat, using yoghurt to reduce the cream and with added peas and chickpeas to bulk it up.

SERVES 4 • 10 MINS, PLUS 30 MINS MARINATING • 25 MINS •

100g natural yoghurt

4 garlic cloves, crushed

1 tbsp grated fresh ginger

1 tbsp tikka masala curry paste

¼ tsp salt

4 skinless, boneless chicken breasts, cut into 3cm chunks

200g frozen peas

500g cooked brown rice, to serve

100ml single cream

50g natural yoghurt

Handful of fresh coriander, roughly chopped, to garnish

FOR THE TIKKA MASALA SAUCE

1 tbsp vegetable oil

2 onions, finely diced

6 tbsp tikka masala curry paste

2 tbsp tomato purée

1 x 500g jar passata

1 x 400g tin chickpeas, drained and rinsed

150ml water

1. First marinate the chicken. Combine the yoghurt, garlic, ginger, curry paste and salt in a medium bowl. Add the chicken chunks and stir to coat. Cover and leave to marinate in the fridge for at least 30 minutes or up to 24 hours.

2. When you're ready to cook, preheat the oven to 250°C/230°C fan/475°F/gas mark 9 and line a baking tray with baking paper.

3. While the oven heats, start the sauce. Heat the oil in a large pan over a medium heat. Add the onions and cook, stirring occasionally, until softened and starting to brown, 5–7 minutes. Add the curry paste and tomato purée. Stir for 1 minute then add the passata, chickpeas and water. Bring to the boil then turn down to simmer for 15–20 minutes so the sauce can thicken and the flavours can develop.

4. Meanwhile, spread the marinated chicken pieces out over the lined baking tray. Bake for 10–15 minutes, turning the chicken halfway through, until they're lightly charred and cooked through.

5. To the sauce, add the cooked chicken and frozen peas. Stir over a low heat for a minute so the peas can defrost. Remove from the heat and allow to cool slightly then stir in the cream and the 50g of natural yoghurt.

6. Serve with the brown rice, garnished with the fresh coriander.

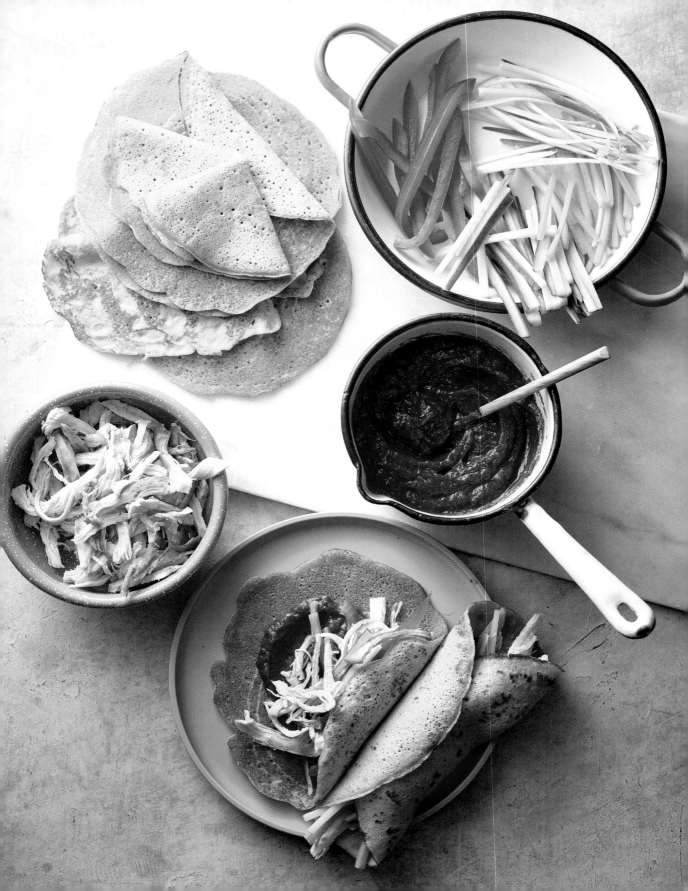

Chicken Pancakes with Plum Sauce

A lighter take on duck pancakes; chicken is a leaner, cheaper meat, and this plum sauce has a boost of fibre and dates that sweeten the sauce without the added sugar of bought versions.

SERVES 4 • 20 MINS • 25 MINS •

FOR THE PANCAKE BATTER

100g carrot, coarsely grated

2 eggs

150g plain white flour

250g milk

½ tbsp vegetable oil

FOR THE SHREDDED CHICKEN

1 tbsp vegetable oil

3 skinless and boneless chicken breasts

200ml chicken stock

FOR THE PLUM SAUCE

100g pitted dates, soaked in boiling water for 10 minutes

½ banana shallot or small onion, finely diced

1 ripe plum, pitted, roughly chopped

2 tbsp orange juice

1 tsp apple cider vinegar

1 tsp soy sauce

½ tsp Chinese five spice

TO SERVE

1 cucumber, cut into matchsticks

1 carrot, cut into matchsticks

1 pepper, deseeded and thinly sliced

4 spring onions, thinly sliced

1. Blitz the pancake ingredients, except the oil, in a blender until smooth. Heat a medium non-stick frying pan over a medium heat and brush with a thin layer of oil. Pour in 60ml of batter and swirl to make a thin crepe. Leave to cook until golden underneath, then flip and repeat on the other side. Remove and repeat with the remaining batter.

2. Prepare the chicken filling. Heat the oil in a medium, non-stick frying pan over a medium heat. Once hot, add the chicken and cook for 3–4 minutes on each side, until golden. Add the stock, cover the pan, and simmer for 5–8 minutes, until the chicken is cooked through. Remove to a board and shred with 2 forks.

3. For the plum sauce, drain the soaked dates and add to a small pan with the remaining sauce ingredients. Cook over a low heat, stirring often, until the plums have softened – around 5 minutes. If the pan is looking too dry, add a splash of water. Remove from the heat and blitz until smooth.

4. Serve the pancakes with the plum sauce, shredded chicken, cucumber, carrot, pepper and spring onions.

Pulled Chicken Burgers

For summery days when you want something lighter, this easy burger is a simple version of the pulled pork classic, using leaner chicken and homemade barbecue sauce, that's lower in sugar.

SERVES 4–6 • 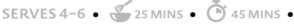 25 MINS • 45 MINS •

1 tbsp olive oil

2 onions, diced

2 x 400g tins chopped tomatoes

4 ripe peaches, stones removed, roughly chopped

3 tbsp dark brown sugar

2 tbsp apple cider vinegar

4 tsp smoked paprika

2 tsp ground cumin

1 tsp ground cinnamon

1 tsp Worcestershire sauce

½ tsp chilli powder

4 boneless, skinless chicken breasts

4 wholemeal burger buns or crusty rolls

2 limes, cut into wedges

FOR THE SLAW

¼ head white cabbage, very thinly shredded

1 medium carrot, coarsely grated

1 small red onion or 1 shallot, thinly sliced

Pinch of salt

3 tbsp natural yoghurt

1 tbsp mayonnaise

1 tsp lemon juice or apple cider vinegar

1. In a large pan, heat the oil over a medium heat and cook the onions until softened and browning, 7–10 minutes. Stir in the tomatoes, peaches, sugar, vinegar, paprika, cumin, cinnamon, Worcestershire sauce and chilli powder. Bring to the boil then turn down to simmer. Add the chicken and simmer for 30 minutes, until cooked through.

2. Remove the chicken to a board, leave the sauce cooking over a low heat, stirring occasionally, until reduced to a thick, dark sauce – around 15 minutes. If you like, you can blitz the sauce with a hand blender off the heat to make it smoother.

3. Shred the chicken using 2 forks and stir a few tablespoons of the tomato sauce into the meat.

4. For the slaw, add the cabbage, carrot and onion to a bowl. Add a pinch of salt and scrunch everything together for a minute to soften the cabbage. Leave for 5 minutes, then pour off any excess liquid. Stir in the yoghurt, mayo and lemon juice.

5. Serve the buns with the shredded chicken, slaw, extra tomato sauce and some lime wedges.

TIP
Any leftover tomato sauce can be frozen in an airtight container for up to 3 months.

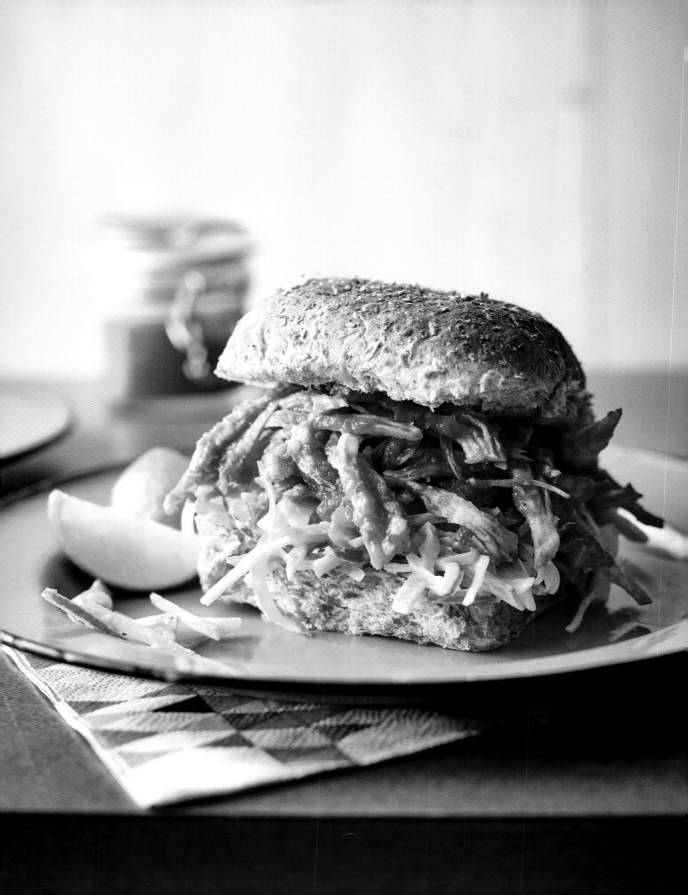

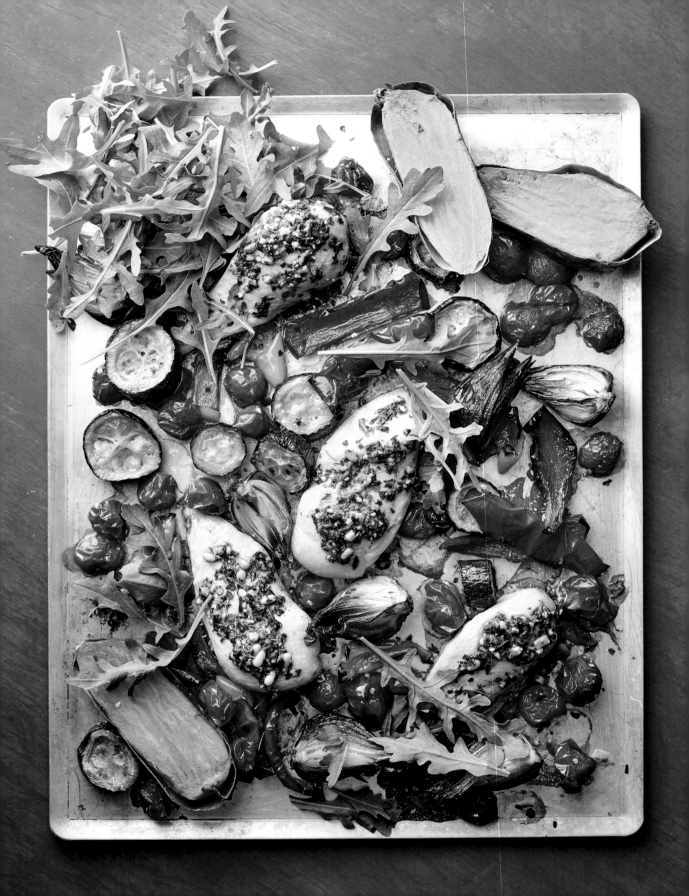

Chicken & Mediterranean Roasted Veg

Easy one-pot dinner that cooks slowly, filling the kitchen with Mediterranean aromas. Vibrant and colourful, it combines chicken with a variety of veg and the herby-garlic flavours of pesto.

SERVES 4 • 20 MINS • 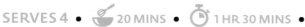 1 HR 30 MINS •

4 medium sweet potatoes

2 peppers, deseeded, cut into 2-cm slices

2 courgettes, cut into 2-cm coins

300g cherry tomatoes

2 red onions, quartered

1 tbsp olive oil

Pinch of salt

4 chicken breast fillets

2 tbsp basil pesto

½ tsp chilli flakes

60g rocket leaves

1. Preheat the oven to 200°C/180°C fan/400°F/gas mark 6. Arrange the oven racks so you have one in the bottom third of the oven and one in the middle third.

2. Prick the sweet potatoes a few times with a fork and place on a baking tray. Set on the lower rack in the oven and bake for 40–45 minutes until tender.

3. Toss the sliced peppers, courgettes, cherry tomatoes and onions with the oil and salt on a separate, large baking tray. Place in the middle third of the oven and bake for 20 minutes. Remove and stir the vegetables. Lay the chicken breasts on the tray and spread the pesto over the chicken, then sprinkle with the chilli flakes. Return the tray to the oven for 20–25 minutes, until the chicken breasts are cooked through.

4. Serve the chicken with the roasted vegetables, baked sweet potatoes and a handful of rocket.

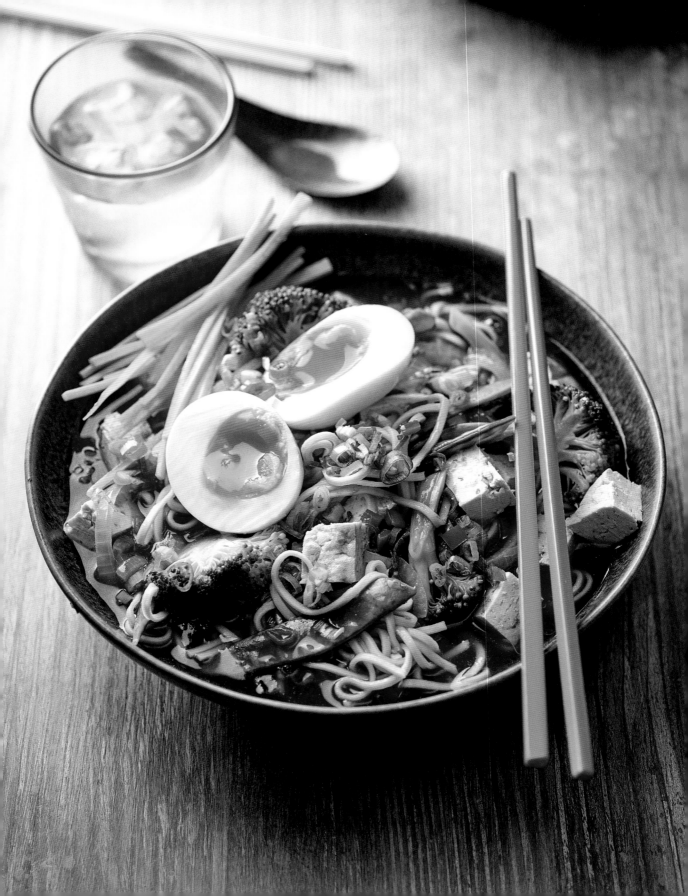

Beef Broth & Broccoli Noodle Soup

A brilliant speedy dinner option that uses plenty of fresh vegetables and protein-packed tofu and eggs to make a warming beef broth. You can add any veg you have in the fridge to this.

SERVES 4 • 15 MINS, PLUS 30 MINS FOR THE TOFU • 22 MINS •

225g smoked tofu

1 tbsp olive oil

1 tsp sesame oil

1 onion, sliced

1 red chilli, deseeded and finely diced

2 tsp grated fresh ginger

4 garlic cloves, crushed

1½ litres water

2 tbsp soy sauce

1 tsp apple cider vinegar

1 beef stock cube

1 small head broccoli, cut into small florets

250g dry, medium egg noodles

200g mangetout

4 eggs

2 carrots, cut into matchsticks or peeled into ribbons, to garnish

2 spring onions, thinly sliced, to garnish

Hot sauce, to serve

1. Drain the tofu then wrap in a clean tea towel and place onto a board. Place another board on top and weigh down with a few books. Set aside for 30 minutes – this allows the excess water to be gently removed from the tofu. Unwrap and cut the tofu into 3cm chunks.

2. Heat both the oils in a large pan over a medium–low heat. Add the onion and cook until starting to turn golden, 7–10 minutes. Add the chilli, ginger and garlic to the pan and cook for 1–2 minutes more until fragrant. Add the water to the pan with the soy sauce, vinegar and stock cube. Bring to the boil then add the broccoli and egg noodles – if the noodles aren't fully submerged, add another 250ml of water to cover them. Cook for 4 minutes until the noodles have softened, then stir in the mangetout and tofu chunks.

3. Gently lower the eggs into a small pan of simmering water. Boil for 6 minutes, remove the eggs from the pan into a colander and hold under cold running water to stop them cooking. Once cool enough to handle, peel and cut the eggs into halves.

4. Divide the broth between 4 bowls and garnish with the halved eggs, the carrots and spring onions. Serve with hot sauce, as needed.

TIP
If you can't find smoked tofu, use plain, firm tofu instead.

Lighter Lasagne

One for a slow day, and the ragu is perfect for batch cooking and freezing. The lentils reduce the amount of meat needed here and increase the fibre content while reducing fat.

SERVES 8 • 30 MINS • 1 HR 20 MINS • ❄

250–300g dried lasagne sheets

FOR THE RAGU

2 tbsp olive oil

4 carrots, diced

2 peppers, deseeded and diced

2 celery sticks, diced

2 onions, diced

600g mushrooms, sliced

250g 5% fat beef mince

2 x 400g tins chopped tomatoes

1 beef stock cube

1 tbsp finely chopped rosemary leaves

120g dry green lentils

Salt

FOR THE CHEESE SAUCE

50g olive oil

75g plain flour

750ml semi-skimmed milk

1 bay leaf

75g mature Cheddar cheese

1. To make the ragu, heat the oil in a large pan over a medium heat and cook the carrots, peppers, celery and onions, stirring occasionally, until softened – around 10 minutes. Remove to a plate and return the pan to the heat.

2. Add the mushrooms with a pinch of salt and cook, stirring, until they've released their liquid and have started to brown. Add to the cooked veg plate.

3. Add the beef to the pan and cook, breaking it into pieces. Add the cooked veg with the tomatoes. Fill each tomato tin with water and pour in, along with the stock cube, rosemary and lentils. Bring to the boil, then simmer. Cover and cook for 30–40 minutes, stirring every 10 minutes, until the lentils are tender.

4. Meanwhile, make the cheese sauce. Heat the oil in a pan over a medium heat, add the flour and stir to a paste. Cook for 2 minutes, stirring, then whisk in the milk, until it is all incorporated and the sauce is smooth. Add the bay leaf and simmer for 5 minutes. Remove from the heat, stir in the cheese and a pinch of salt.

5. Ten minutes before the ragu is ready, preheat the oven to 200°C/180°C fan/400°F/gas mark 6. Then assemble the lasagne. Discard the bay leaf. Spread some ragu sauce over the bottom of a 23 x 33cm baking dish. Top with a layer of lasagne. Spread a third of the ragu on top, followed by a third of the cheese sauce. Repeat twice, finishing with cheese sauce.

6. Bake for 30–40 minutes until browned on top. Cool for 10 minutes before cutting and serving.

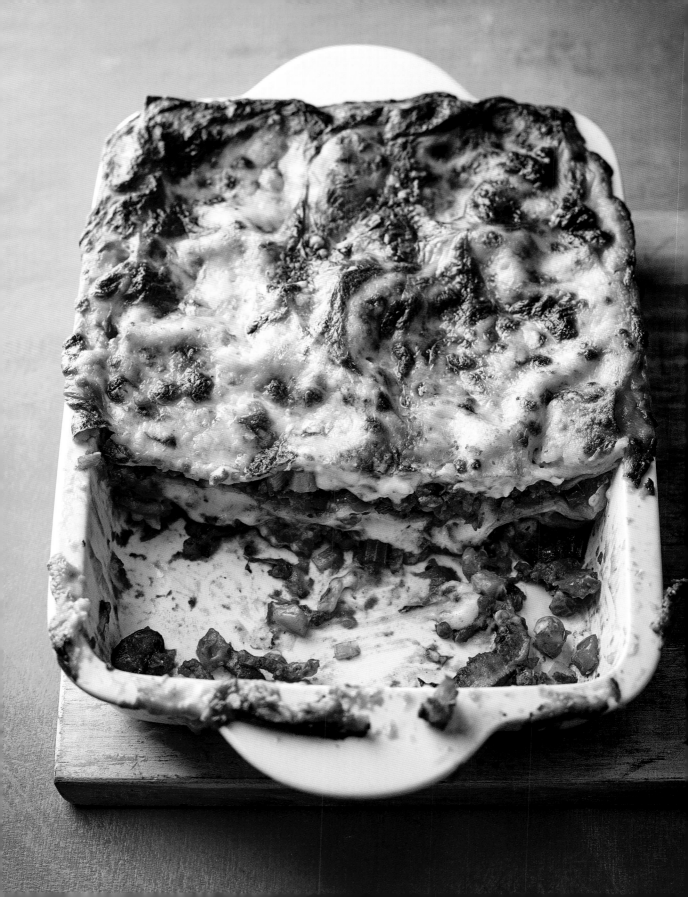

Shepherd's Pie

Simple twists on a family favourite make this a fibre- and protein-packed version. Cannellini beans add a creamy touch to the mash, while lentils bulk out the meat sauce. Good for freezing.

SERVES 4–6 • 25 MINS • 1 HR 20 MINS • ❄

1 tbsp olive oil

4 celery sticks, diced

3 onions, diced

2 medium carrots, diced

250g lamb mince

120g tomato purée

1 beef stock cube

1½ litres water

200g red lentils

1 tbsp Worcestershire sauce

1 tbsp finely chopped rosemary

400g floury potatoes, e.g. Maris Piper, quartered

2 x 400g tins cannellini beans, drained

2 tbsp extra virgin olive oil

Salt and freshly ground black pepper

1. Preheat the oven to 200°C/180°C fan/400°F/gas mark 6.

2. Heat the oil in a large pan over a medium heat. Add the celery, onions and carrots and cook, stirring occasionally, until softened – around 10 minutes. Remove the vegetables to a plate and add the lamb mince to the pan. Cook until no longer pink, then stir in the tomato purée, beef stock cube and water. Bring to the boil then stir in the lentils, Worcestershire sauce and rosemary. Simmer for 20–30 minutes, adding a bit more water to the pan if it looks dry, until the lentils are cooked through. Tip the mixture into a 23 x 33cm baking dish.

3. While the meat is cooking, place the potatoes into a medium pan and cover with cold water. Bring to the boil, then turn down to simmer and cook until tender, around 15 minutes. Drain the potatoes, return them to the pan and mash lightly.

4. Drain the cannellini beans but reserve around 100ml of the liquid from their tins. Add the drained beans to the pan of mashed potatoes along with the olive oil. Mash, loosening with the reserved liquid from the cannellini bean tins as needed to get a soft, smooth mash. Season with salt and pepper to taste. Dot the mash over the mixture in the baking dish and spread out to cover the surface. Bake for 30–40 minutes until the filling is bubbling and the mash is slightly golden.

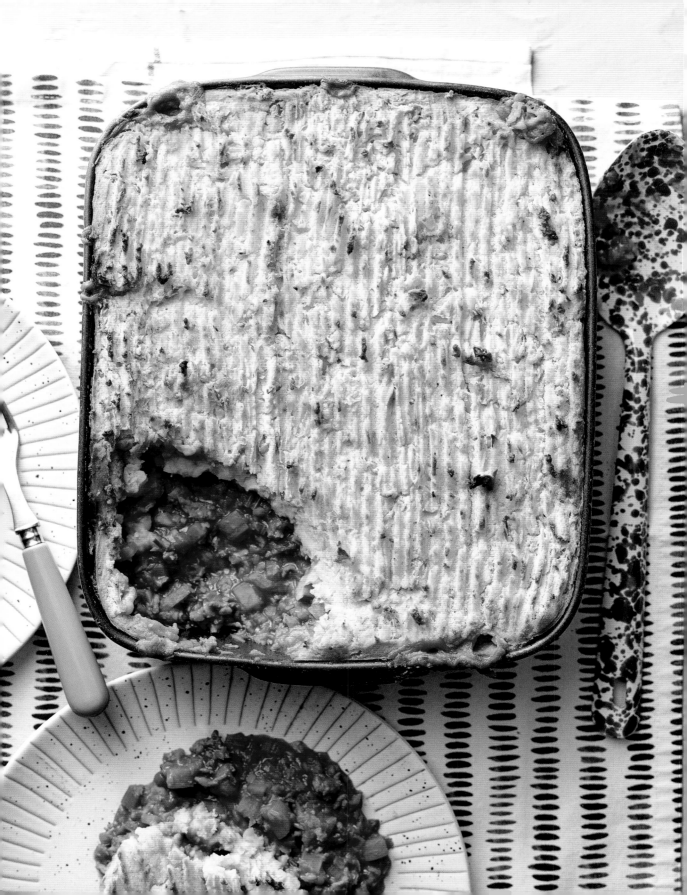

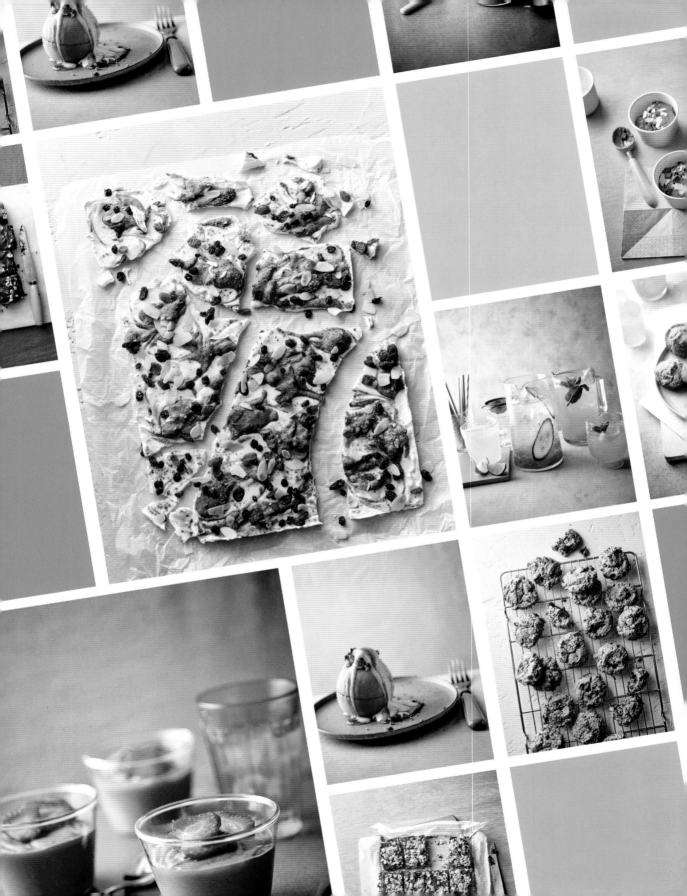

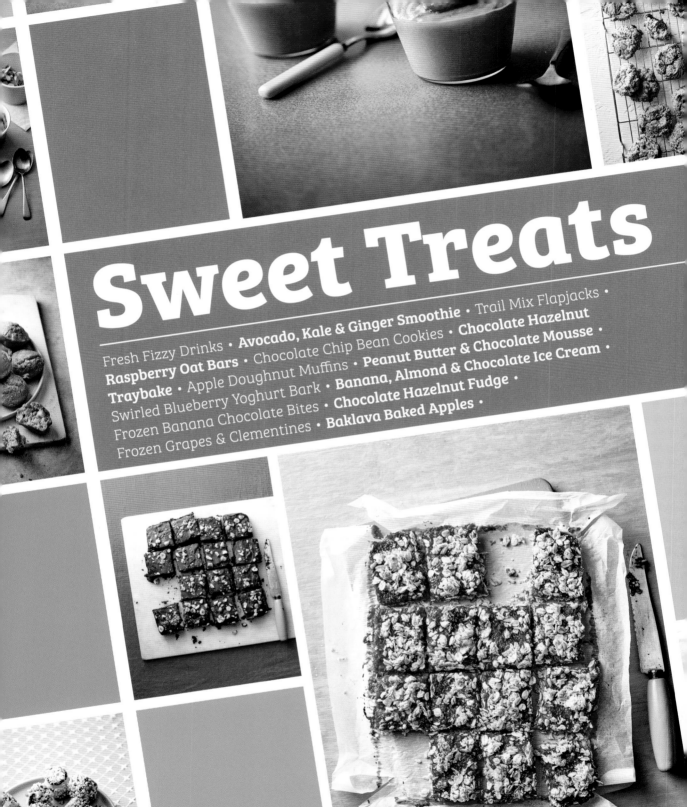

Sweet Treats

Fresh Fizzy Drinks • **Avocado, Kale & Ginger Smoothie** • Trail Mix Flapjacks •
Raspberry Oat Bars • Chocolate Chip Bean Cookies • **Chocolate Hazelnut**
Traybake • Apple Doughnut Muffins • **Peanut Butter & Chocolate Mousse** •
Swirled Blueberry Yoghurt Bark • **Chocolate Hazelnut Ice Cream** •
Frozen Banana Chocolate Bites • **Chocolate Hazelnut Fudge** •
Frozen Grapes & Clementines • **Baklava Baked Apples** •

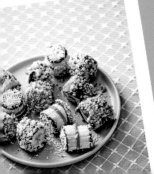

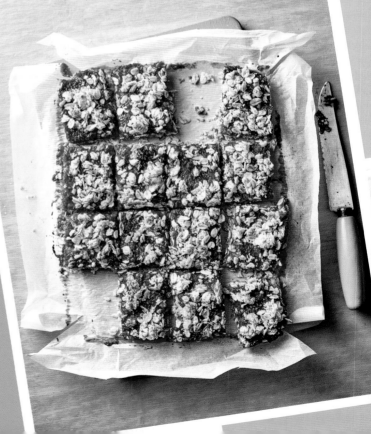

Fresh Fizzy Drinks

Keep hydrated with these low-sugar but delicious alternatives to artificially sweetened fizzy drinks. Full of natural herb and fruit flavours that are particularly refreshing on a warm day.

MAKES 4–6 • 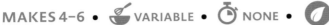 VARIABLE • NONE •

Green Tea, Mint & Lemon Cooler

4 green tea bags

4 sprigs of fresh mint, plus extra to garnish (optional)

5 strips of lemon zest, plus wedges to garnish (optional)

4 tbsp lemon juice

500ml boiling water

1½ litres cold water

Ice cubes, to serve

1. Place the tea bags, mint, lemon zest and juice into a jug. Pour over the boiling water and leave to steep for 2 minutes. Remove the tea bags and top up with the cold water. Pour into a glass with some ice cubes and garnish with lemon wedges and mint sprigs, if you like.

Ginger, Lime & Orange Fizz

20g fresh ginger, finely grated

50ml orange juice

Juice of 1 lime, plus slices to garnish (optional)

2 litres sparkling water

Ice cubes, to serve

1. Mix together the grated ginger, orange and lime juices in a small bowl then press through a sieve to remove solids, catching the liquid in a jug.

2. Top up with the sparkling water and add some ice cubes. Serve garnished with lime slices, if you like.

Strawberry & Cucumber Cooler

100g strawberries, hulled, plus slices to garnish (optional)

10 slices cucumber

2 tbsp lemon juice

2 litres sparkling water

50ml apple juice (optional)

Ice cubes, to serve

1. Mash the strawberries with the back of a fork. Scrape into a jug then mix in the cucumber slices and lemon juice. Pour in the sparkling water. Taste – if you want it a bit sweeter, add the apple juice and mix again.

2. Serve with ice, garnished with a strawberry slice, if you like.

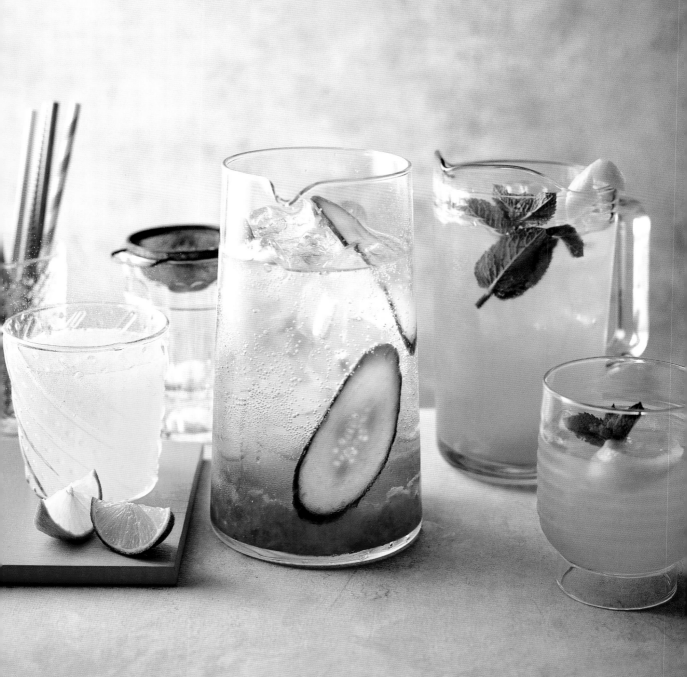

Avocado, Kale & Ginger Smoothie

This creamy smoothie is a delicious way to start the day, with nutritious greens and slow-release energy from the avocado. Hemp seeds are optional, but add healthy fats like omega 3.

SERVES 4 • 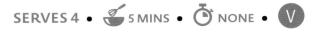 5 MINS • NONE • V

50g chopped curly kale

150g frozen pineapple chunks

125ml skimmed milk or plant-based milk

125ml water

½ ripe avocado, peeled and stoned

2 tbsp lemon juice

10g fresh ginger

2 tbsp hemp seed (optional)

2 pitted dates (optional)

1. Blitz everything, apart from the seeds and dates, if using, together in a blender until completely smooth. Taste and, if you want it a bit sweeter, add more pineapple or add the dates and seeds and blitz again until smooth.

Trail Mix Flapjacks

These fruity, nutty flapjacks make a delicious snack, and are perfect for popping into lunchboxes. Full of slow-release energy, these will keep your blood sugar levels in balance.

MAKES 16 SQUARES • **20 MINS, PLUS 10 MINS SOAKING** • **20 MINS** •

100g dried fruit, any larger types roughly chopped

80g golden syrup

60ml vegetable oil

200g jumbo oats

70g wholemeal flour

½ tsp baking powder

2 eggs

100g mixed seeds and nuts, roughly chopped

100g dark chocolate (70–85% cocoa), roughly chopped

1. Preheat the oven to 200°C/180°C fan/400°F/gas mark 6 and line a 23cm square cake tin with baking paper.

2. Place the dried fruit into a medium bowl and cover with boiling water. Set aside for 10 minutes to soften, then drain well.

3. In a medium pan, stir together the golden syrup and vegetable oil over a medium-low heat until it starts to gently bubble. Remove from the heat and add the oats, flour, baking powder and eggs. Mix together until combined, then fold in the drained dried fruit, seeds and nuts and chocolate.

4. Scrape the mixture into the prepared cake tin and press down to fill the tin and form an even layer. Bake for 12–15 minutes until the edges are looking slightly golden and the flapjacks are soft but not sticky.

5. Allow to cool then slice into 16 squares. Store in an airtight container for up to 5 days.

Raspberry Oat Bars

A sticky, fruity, delicious alternative to a snack bar, these are lower in sugar than anything you can buy, and are easy to make. Perfect for snacking on or as a treat in a lunchbox.

MAKES 16 SQUARES • **20 MINS** • **25 MINS** •

40g unsalted butter

20g olive oil

4 tbsp golden syrup

210g jumbo oats

25g sunflower seeds, roughly chopped

2 tbsp wholemeal plain flour

1 egg white

200g frozen raspberries

1. Preheat the oven to 200°C/180°C fan/400°F/gas mark 6 and line a 20cm square cake tin with baking paper.

2. Melt the butter, oil and 3 tablespoons of golden syrup in a medium pan. Once melted, remove from the heat and stir in the oats, sunflower seeds and flour until coated. Finally, mix in the egg white. Crumble two-thirds of this mixture into the prepared cake tin and press down into an even layer.

3. Combine the frozen raspberries and remaining 1 tablespoon of golden syrup in a small pan. Place over a low heat and cook until the raspberries have defrosted and the mixture has started to bubble. Take off the heat and pour over the oat crust in the tin. Crumble the remaining oat mixture over the raspberry jam.

4. Bake for 20 minutes until golden. Allow to cool in the tin, then cut into 16 squares. Store in an airtight container in the fridge for up to 3 days or freeze for up to 3 months.

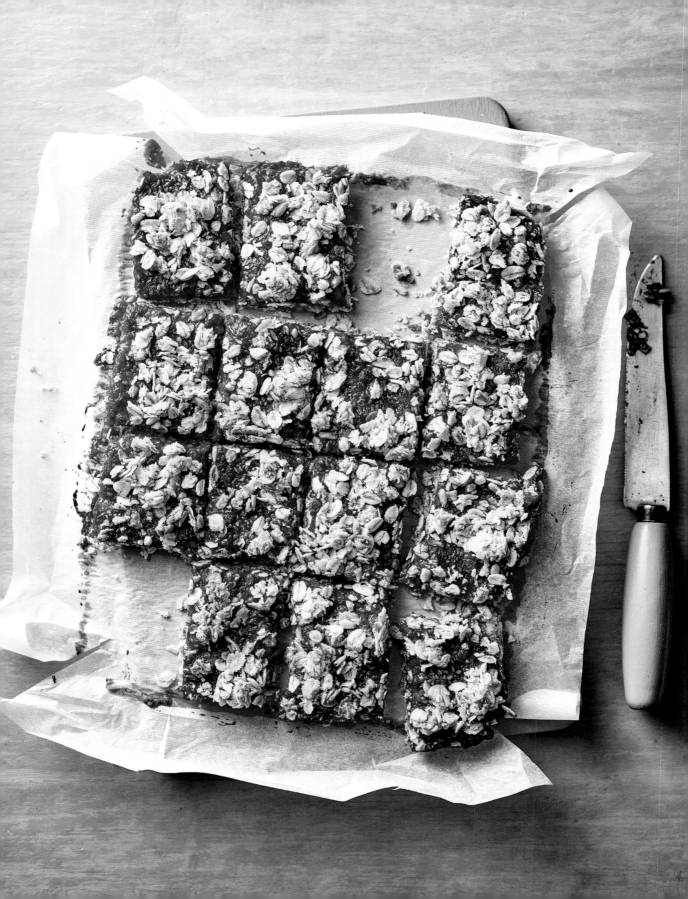

Chocolate Chip Bean Cookies

Beans might sound a strange addition to a cookie, but they provide protein and fibre and you can't taste them. The butter, sugar and chocolate chunks lend a more traditional cookie flavour.

MAKES 20 • 15 MINS • 12 MINS • **V**

50g porridge oats

100g light brown sugar

50g ground almonds

45g unsalted butter

1 x 400g tin cannellini beans, drained and rinsed

65g peanut butter

1 tsp vanilla extract

½ tsp bicarbonate of soda

¼ tsp salt

100g dark chocolate (70–85% cocoa), roughly chopped

1. Preheat the oven to 200°C/180°C fan/400°F/gas mark 6 and line two baking trays with baking paper.

2. Blend the oats in a food processor to get a scruffy flour. Add the sugar, almonds and butter and blitz until combined. Add the drained cannellini beans, peanut butter, vanilla, bicarbonate of soda and salt, then blitz until smooth. Add the chopped chocolate to the food processor and pulse twice, just to mix it through.

3. Take heaped tablespoons of the mixture and blob them onto the prepared tray, spacing them a few centimetres apart to allow for spreading in the oven.

4. Bake for 8–12 minutes, until the edges are set but the middles are still soft. Allow to cool on the tray for 1 minute before transferring to a wire rack to cool completely.

5. Store in an airtight container for up to 1 week.

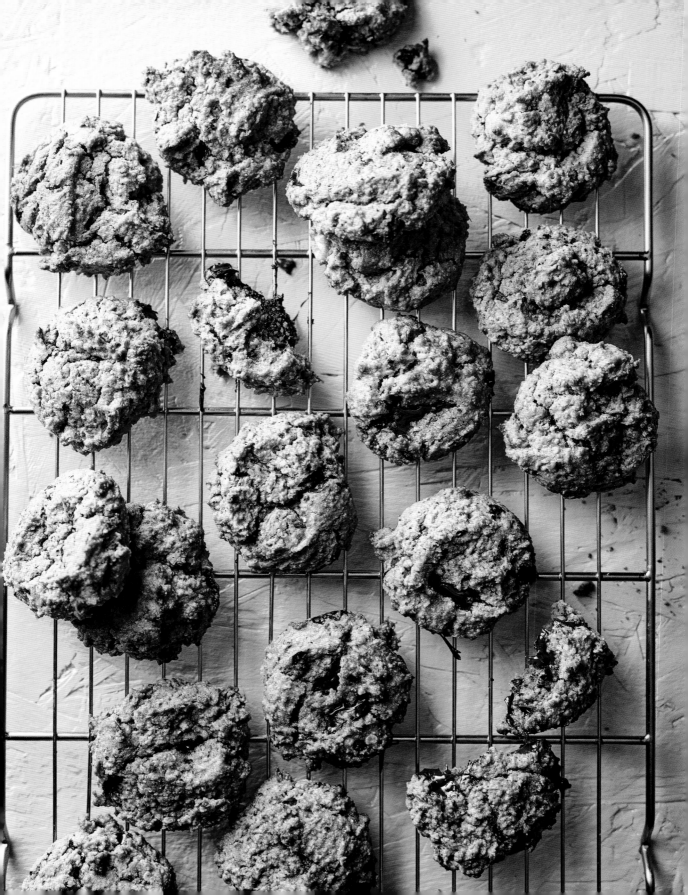

Chocolate Hazelnut Traybake

Black beans here add protein and fibre, helping to reduce sugar spikes and give the traybake a cakey texture, while prunes provide a natural sweetness, so you don't need as much sugar.

MAKES 16 SQUARES • **15 MINS** • **20 MINS** •

100g pitted prunes

1 x 400g tin black beans, drained and rinsed

2 eggs

50ml extra virgin olive oil

50g granulated sugar

70g unsweetened cocoa powder

1 tsp baking powder

2 tsp vanilla extract

Pinch of salt

50g hazelnuts, roughly chopped

50g dark chocolate, roughly chopped

1. Preheat the oven to 200°C/180°C fan/400°F/gas mark 6 and line a 20cm square cake tin with baking paper.

2. Place the prunes into a small bowl and cover with boiling water. Set aside to soak for 5 minutes then drain.

3. Blitz the drained prunes with the black beans, eggs, oil, sugar, cocoa powder, baking powder, vanilla and salt until smooth. Fold in half of the chopped hazelnuts.

4. Scrape the mixture into the prepared cake tin and spread out into an even layer. Bake for 20 minutes, until a toothpick inserted into the centre of the cake comes out clean.

5. Sprinkle the chopped chocolate over the hot cake and leave to sit for 5 minutes for it to melt. Spread the melted chocolate evenly over the top of the cake and sprinkle with the remaining chopped hazelnuts.

6. Cool in the tin, then remove to a wire rack to cool completely. Once cold, cut into 16 squares. Store in an airtight container for up to 5 days.

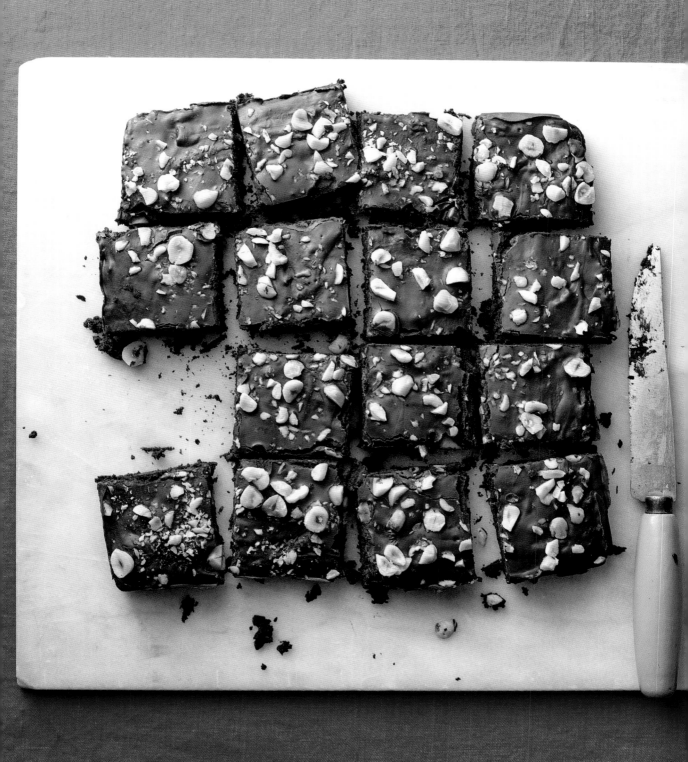

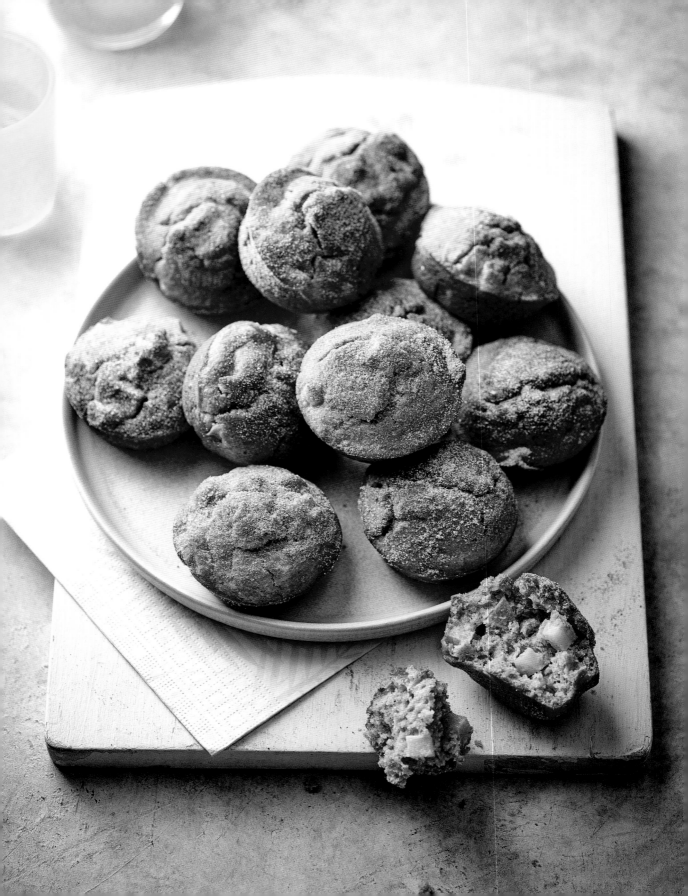

Apple Doughnut Muffins

Healthy eating doesn't mean saying goodbye to all treats (especially these super-healthy homemade versions). Wholemeal flour and apple add fibre, and baking reduces the fat.

MAKES 12 • 15 MINS • 45 MINS • V

3 eating apples, cored

70ml olive oil

50ml milk

50g light brown sugar

2 eggs

180g wholemeal plain flour

40g ground almonds

1½ tsp baking powder

¼ tsp ground nutmeg (optional)

FOR THE CINNAMON SUGAR TOPPING

1 tbsp caster sugar

½ tsp ground cinnamon

1 tbsp butter, melted

1. Preheat the oven to 200°C/180°C fan/400°F/gas mark 6 and grease the wells of a 12-hole muffin tin with a little melted butter.

2. Roughly chop two of the cored apples and add to a medium pan with a splash of water. Cover with a lid and cook over a low heat for 15 minutes until completely soft. Blitz until smooth and set aside. Chop the remaining apple into 1cm chunks and set aside.

3. Measure 150g of the puréed apple into a medium bowl. Add the olive oil, milk, sugar and eggs then mix together until smooth. Add the flour, ground almonds, baking powder, nutmeg and apple chunks then fold together until just combined.

4. Divide between the wells and bake for 25–30 minutes until golden on top and a toothpick inserted into the centre of the muffins comes out clean. Run a knife around the edge of each muffin to loosen then tip out onto a wire rack.

5. Make the topping by combining the caster sugar and ground cinnamon in a small bowl. Brush the tops of the warm muffins with the melted butter and sprinkle with the cinnamon sugar. These are best eaten the day they're made or can be kept in an airtight container for up to 3 days.

Peanut Butter & Chocolate Mousse

Peanut butter and chocolate are a match made in heaven, and here the nut butter adds healthy fats and a creamy texture, with the cream replaced by more nutritious tofu.

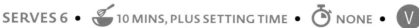 SERVES 6 • 10 MINS, PLUS SETTING TIME • NONE • V

100g dark chocolate, melted
220g silken tofu
40g smooth peanut butter
2 egg whites
200g strawberries, hulled and sliced

1. Blitz together the melted chocolate, silken tofu and peanut butter until smooth.

2. Place the egg whites into a large, clean bowl and whisk with electric beaters until you get stiff peaks.

3. Pour the chocolate mixture into the bowl of beaten egg whites and gently fold together until no white streaks remain, being careful not to knock out too much air.

4. Divide the mixture between 6 small glasses or bowls and set in the fridge for at least 1 hour until set. These will keep in the fridge for up to 2 days.

5. When ready to serve, top with the sliced strawberries.

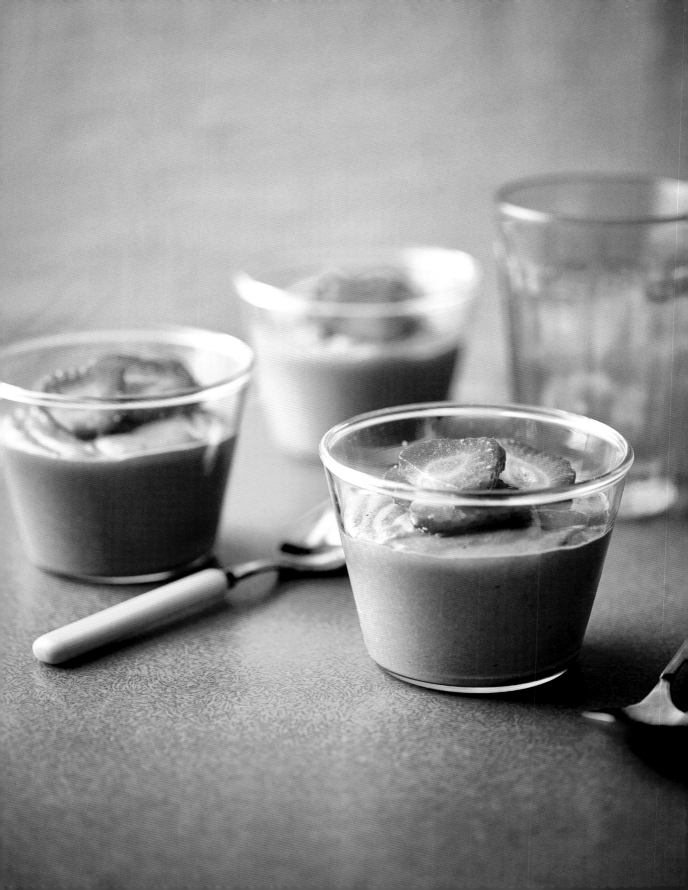

Swirled Blueberry Yoghurt Bark

These gorgeous-coloured pieces of yoghurt bark make a delicious and cheerful treat. Yoghurt provides essential calcium and protein, making these a great snack to keep you fuller longer.

SERVES 4–6 • 5 MINS, PLUS 2 HRS FREEZING • 5 MINS •

100g frozen blueberries

300g Greek yoghurt

20g flaked almonds or chopped almonds

1 tsp flaxseeds

50g dried fruit (if using any larger dried fruits, roughly chop them first)

1. Cook the blueberries in a small, lidded pot over a low heat until defrosted and soft – around 5 minutes. Mash with a potato masher or the back of a fork into a chunky purée. Allow to cool.

2. Mix the yoghurt so it loosens up a bit. Spread 200g of the yoghurt onto a lined tray. To the remaining yoghurt, mix in the cooled blueberry compote. Dot this over the surface of the yoghurt on the tray and swirl together. Sprinkle on the almonds, flaxseeds and dried fruit.

3. Freeze for 2 hours or until solid, then break into shards and eat. Store the extra pieces in an airtight container in the freezer for up to 2 weeks.

TIPS

Use whatever nuts and seeds you like here, or even bits of granola (page 70).

You can make the purée using any other berry you like, just follow the same recipe.

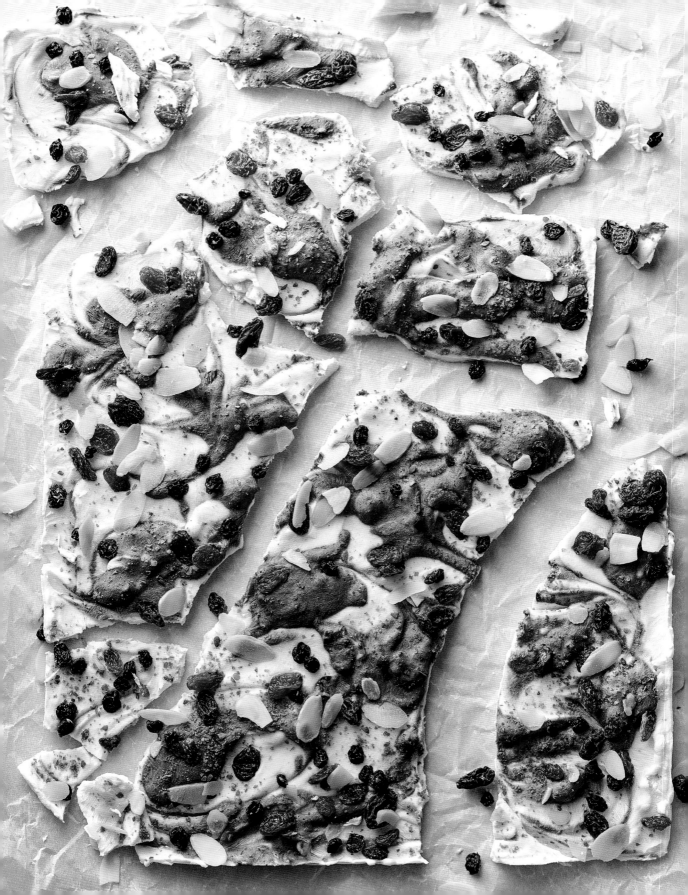

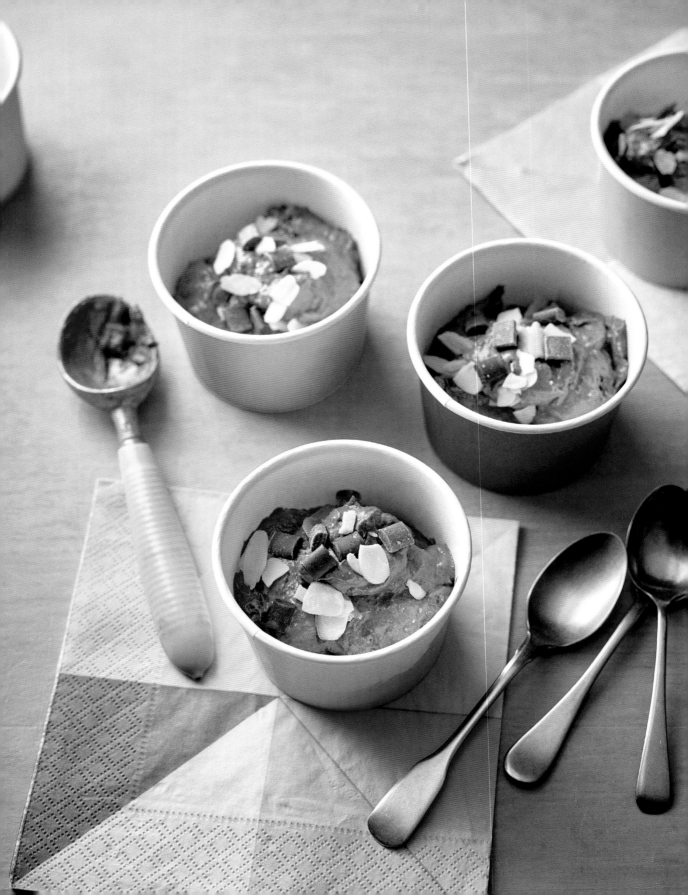

Banana, Almond & Chocolate Ice Cream

Such a simple way to make ice cream; frozen banana is easily blended into a creamy, smooth ice-cream texture, pepped up with the flavours and crunch of chocolate chips and almonds.

SERVES 4 • 10 MINS, PLUS FREEZING • 2 MINS •

20g flaked almonds

3 large, ripe bananas (peeled weight 350g)

2 tbsp smooth almond butter

1 tbsp milk or non-dairy milk

1 tsp vanilla extract

2 tbsp unsweetened cocoa powder

2 tbsp chocolate chips

1. Place the flaked almonds into a small frying pan over a medium–low heat. Toast, stirring often, until golden and fragrant, around 2 minutes, then tip out onto a plate and set aside.

2. Peel the bananas and cut into roughly 2cm thick chunks. Lay onto a lined baking tray and freeze until solid, around 1 hour.

3. Tip the frozen banana slices into a food processor and blitz until they start to break down into very small pieces. Add the almond butter, milk and vanilla and blend until smooth – you may need to stop the food processor to scrape down the sides a few times. Add the cocoa powder and blend to combine.

4. You can serve the ice cream immediately, sprinkled with the toasted almonds and chocolate chips, if you like a soft-serve texture. For a firmer ice cream, fold in the toasted almonds and chocolate chips then transfer to a loaf tin or small freezerproof container and freeze for 1–2 hours until firm enough to scoop. (If frozen for longer than 2 hours the ice cream will need to thaw for 10 minutes before serving and will likely have a slightly icy texture.)

Frozen Banana Chocolate Bites

These little bites will satisfy any craving for a sweet treat. Creamy frozen banana is rolled in protein- and healthy fat-packed nut butter and drizzled with heart-healthy dark chocolate.

SERVES 2–4 • 10 MINS, PLUS FREEZING • NONE •

2 large ripe bananas, sliced into 1-cm coins

60g almond butter or nut butter of choice

½ tsp ground cinnamon

1 tsp extra virgin olive oil

50g dark chocolate (70–85% cocoa), melted

30g chopped nuts, e.g. hazelnuts, pistachios, walnuts, desiccated coconut

1. Lay half of the banana slices onto a baking tray lined with baking paper.

2. Mix the nut butter and cinnamon in a small bowl until smooth. Spoon a bit less than ½ teaspoon of nut butter onto each of the banana slices on the tray. Top with a second slice of banana, pressing down to squish the nut butter to the edges.

3. Freeze the banana 'sandwiches' for 10 minutes to firm up.

4. Mix the olive oil into the melted chocolate and pour into a small bowl. Place the nuts onto a small plate.

5. Dip the side of each frozen banana sandwich into the melted chocolate then quickly dip into your favourite chopped nuts. Set back onto the lined tray. Repeat with the rest of the banana slices. Place back into the freezer until set, around 5 minutes. Once frozen, pop them into an airtight container and freeze for up to 2 weeks.

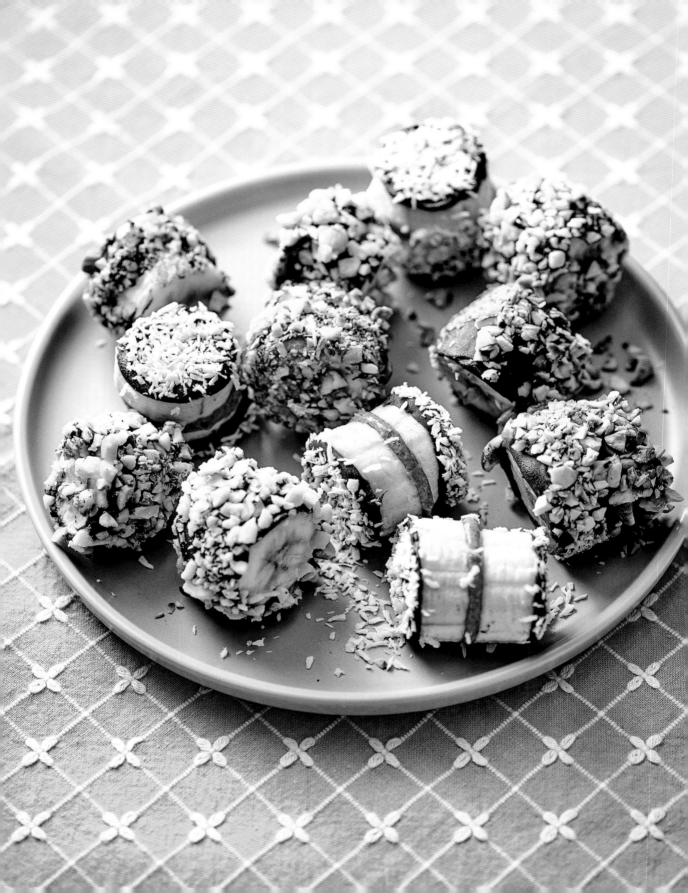

Baklava Baked Apples

A deceptively indulgent treat – baked fresh apples with sweetness provided by dates and honey. A delicious dessert that helps avoid blood sugar spikes.

SERVES 4 • 20 MINS • 25 MINS •

4 eating apples
50g pitted dates
50g walnuts
50g pistachios
30g butter
Zest of 1 lemon
Natural yoghurt, to serve

FOR THE SYRUP
2 tbsp runny honey
Juice of ½ lemon
½ tsp ground cinnamon

1. Preheat the oven to 200°C/180°C fan/400°F/gas mark 6 and line a baking dish with baking paper.

2. Remove the cores from the apples, leaving the bottom 1cm intact – you can use an apple corer for this or a paring knife. Score into the apple skin around the circumference of each apple then set onto the baking dish.

3. Combine the dates, walnuts, pistachios, butter and lemon zest in a food processor and blend until chunkily chopped but not to a paste.

4. Push the mixture into the holes in the apples and scatter any remaining mixture around the apples on the tray.

5. Bake for 10 minutes then remove the excess nut mixture from the tray onto a plate. Return the dish to the oven and cook for a further 10–15 minutes, until the apples are soft but not mushy. Place onto individual dishes and scatter over the extra nut mixture.

6. For the syrup, heat the honey, lemon juice and cinnamon in a small pan over a low heat until it just starts to bubble. Remove from the heat and pour some over each baked apple. Serve with the natural yoghurt.

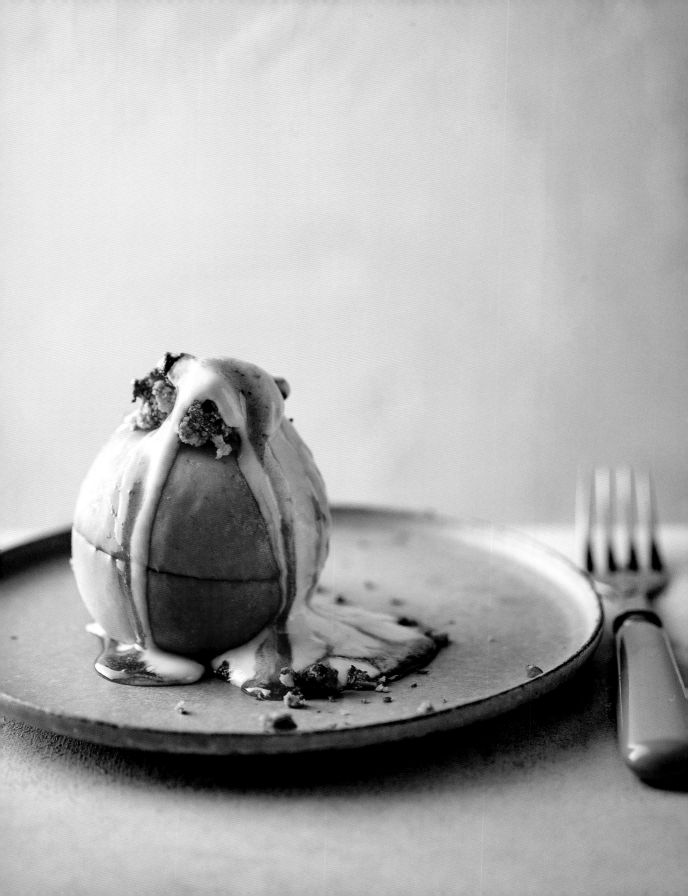

Cooks' Notes

Key to cooking symbols

 Vegetarian   Vegan   Freezable

 Prep time   Cook time

General

Eggs are medium unless stated otherwise.
Always wash fresh produce before cooking.

Approximate liquid conversions

Metric	Imperial
50ml	2fl oz
125ml	4fl oz
175ml	6fl oz
225ml	8fl oz
300ml	10fl oz/½ pint
450ml	16fl oz
600ml	20fl oz/1 pint
1 litre	35fl oz/1¾ pints

Spoon measures

Spoon measurements are level unless otherwise specified.

· 1 teaspoon (tsp) = 5ml
· 1 tablespoon (tbsp) = 15ml

Oven temperatures

°C	Fan	°F	Gas
140	120	275	1
150	130	300	2
170	150	325	3
180	160	350	4
190	170	375	5
200	180	400	6
220	200	425	7
230	210	450	8
240	220	475	9

Weekly Meal Planner

MONDAY

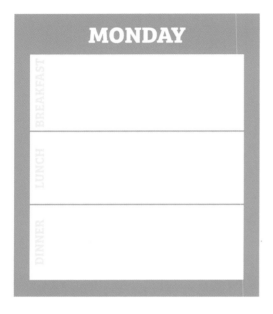

BREAKFAST

LUNCH

DINNER

TUESDAY

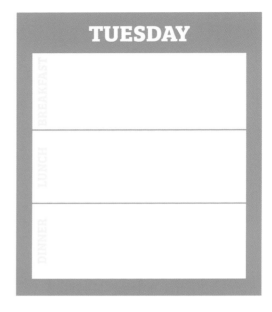

BREAKFAST

LUNCH

DINNER

WEDNESDAY

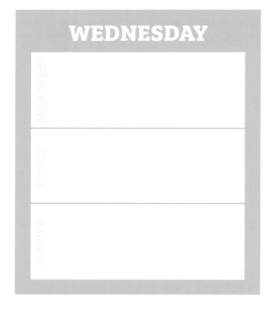

BREAKFAST

LUNCH

DINNER

THURSDAY

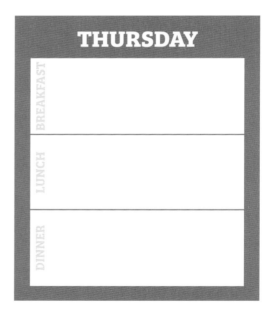

BREAKFAST

LUNCH

DINNER

FRIDAY

BREAKFAST

LUNCH

DINNER

SATURDAY

BREAKFAST

LUNCH

DINNER

SUNDAY

BREAKFAST

LUNCH

DINNER

NOTES/SNACKS

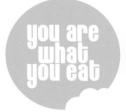
you are what you eat

Weekly Meal Planner

MONDAY

BREAKFAST

LUNCH

DINNER

TUESDAY

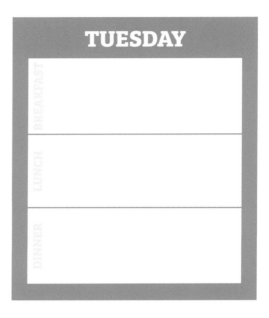

WEDNESDAY

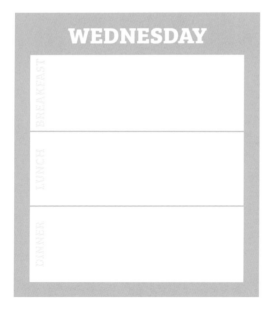

THURSDAY

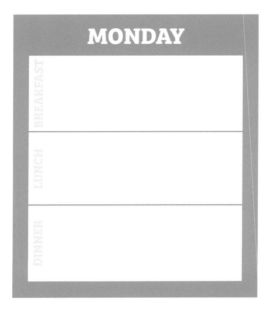

BREAKFAST

LUNCH

DINNER

FRIDAY

BREAKFAST

LUNCH

DINNER

SATURDAY

BREAKFAST

LUNCH

DINNER

SUNDAY

BREAKFAST

LUNCH

DINNER

NOTES/SNACKS

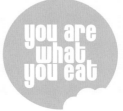
you are
what
you eat

Food Diary

	BREAKFAST	LUNCH	DINNER
M			
T			
W			
T			
F			
S			
S			

SNACKS	NOTES

Acknowledgements

CPL

There is a brilliant team behind the making of *You Are What You Eat*, and our thanks to go all of them and to: Alan Ahmet, Dominique Belcourt, Pete Benn, Jess Blair, Dermot Caulfield, Peter Elphick, Ashley Ganly-Kesington, Jasmine Gurung, Professor Lindsay Hall, Elea Huston, Mark Knowles, Mitchell Langcaster-James, Kate Llewellyn-Waters, Susie Mackie, Dan Marlow, David Miller, Sarah Nightingale, Justine Pattison, Theodore Ross, Liam Royales, Nicole Streak, Matt Tatem, Julia Whitehouse.

And of course a big thank you to our presenters, Trisha Goddard and Dr Amir Khan.

Thanks to all the contributors to the show who have shared their lives and stories with us: Dennica Abdo, Sabrina Ali, Helen Franks, Zoe Gilfillan, Dawn Gledhill, Ryan Gray, Laura Howey, Leonie Napper, John Shevlin, Adam Trunks, Jackie Uphill and Alexandra Webb.

Thank you to Kate Fox at HQ for commissioning this book.

HQ

HQ would like to thank: Toby Scott for photography, Sarah Birks for prop styling, Rosie Reynolds and Troy Willis for food styling; James Gillham for cover photography; Rebecca Woods for cover food styling; Georgie Hewitt for art direction; Andy Chapman and David Macartney at Plum5 for page design; Izy Hossack for recipe work; Helena Caldon for project editing. And thanks to all the team at CPL Productions.

you are
what
you eat

When using kitchen appliances please always follow the manufacturer's instructions.

HQ
An imprint of HarperCollinsPublishers Ltd
1 London Bridge Street
London SE1 9GF
www.harpercollins.co.uk

HarperCollinsPublishers
1st Floor, Watermarque Building, Ringsend Road
Dublin 4, Ireland

10 9 8 7 6 5 4 3 2 1

First published in Great Britain by
HQ, an imprint of HarperCollinsPublishers Ltd 2021

ISBN: 978-0-00-851160-9

This book is published to accompany the television series entitled *You Are What You Eat*
first broadcast on Channel 5 in the UK. *You Are What You Eat* is a CPL Production

This book is produced from independently certified FSC™ paper
to ensure responsible forest management.

For more information visit: www.harpercollins.co.uk/green

Food Photographer: Toby Scott
Page 6: James Gillham © CPL Productions
All other images courtesy © Shutterstock
Art Director: Georgina Hewitt
Designer: Plum5 Ltd
Editorial Director: Kate Fox
Project Editor: Helena Caldon

Printed and bound in Great Britain by
Bell and Bain Ltd, Glasgow

The information in this book will be helpful to most people but is not a substitute for advice from a medical practitioner and is not tailored to individual requirements. You should always check with your doctor before starting an exercise programme, particularly if you have not exercised before. The author and publishers do not accept any responsibility for any injury or adverse effects that may arise from the use or misuse of the information in this book.